ADHD Complex

ADHD Complex

Practicing Mental Health in Primary Care

HARLAN R. GEPHART, MD, FAAP
Clinical Professor of Pediatrics, Emeritus
University of Washington School of Medicine
Seattle, Washington

ELSEVIER

ELSEVIER

3251 Riverport Lane
St. Louis, Missouri 63043

ADHD Complex: Practicing Mental Health in Primary Care   ISBN: 978-0-323-64304-7

Content Strategist: Lauren Boyle
Content Development Manager: Kathy Padilla
Content Development Specialist: Kristi Anderson
Publishing Services Manager: Jameel Shereen
Project Manager: Nadhiya Sekar
Designer: Gopalakrishnan Venkatraman

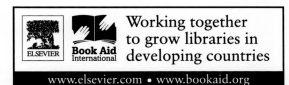

Printed in United States of America

Last digit is the print number: 9 8 7 6 5 4 3 2 1

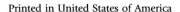

Foreword

It is both a personal and professional pleasure for me to be allowed to write the foreword for this book. It is a personal pleasure, as I have gotten to know Harlan Gephart in our more than 15 years' work together. I have discovered in him an extraordinary, compassionate, and competent human being, as well as a lifelong friend. By his quiet example, from him I have learned much about how to live one's life and "what's most important," and he even has taught me some fly-fishing along the way.

But writing the foreword gives me unmatched professional pleasure as well. Why? In my 35 years of experience in child and adolescent psychiatry clinical practice, training, and research, I have never met another pediatrician with the breadth, depth, and length of experience in helping kids with mental health problems than my good friend Harlan Gephart. A renowned pediatrician, Harlan has truly "seen it done, done it, and got the T-shirt," or in this case multiple T-shirts, jerseys, cleats, and an extensive array of tools and playing equipment that have allowed him to change many children's lives. But this book allows him to expand his impact to the extent that many other pediatric primary care providers can reap from these pages of his lifelong experience and hard-earned clinical wisdom.

Since the founding of The REACH Institute over 10 years ago, I have had the pleasure to work alongside Harlan, a master teacher, as he has shared his treasure trove of experiences and wisdom. Harlan has been one of The REACH Institute's "star" teachers in our trainings of over 2200 practicing primary care clinicians. While his teaching impact has been extraordinary, I realized that his experience and wisdom needed to reach even more clinicians than allowed by The REACH Institute's training programs. So when Harlan decided that he should commit to the pages of a book what he has learned about children's mental health in primary care, I was delighted and honored to be asked to write this foreword.

Primary care providers need the right tools, and I believe that this book is the right tool at the right time. The book is organized by the problems that pediatric primary care clinicians most frequently see: first, ADHD, followed by anxiety, depression, and other common disorders. For each of these areas, Harlan has distilled a wealth of information into the most important *do's* and *don't's*, easily grasped in bullet form, clinical pearls, and other practical tools and strategies based on individual cases that one is likely to encounter.

I have long felt that we needed to "clone" Harlan Gephart, as most children and families need to obtain basic mental health care from their trusted and known primary care provider. This book may be the closest chance that we will get to cloning Dr. Gephart.

So please read it carefully and reread it as you get more experience in delivering mental health services to your pediatric patients. It will not only change your own practice and enrich your clinical life but also allow you to change the lives of many children who otherwise would not receive help.

Thank you, Harlan, for your lifelong dedication to children, and thank you for sharing with your colleagues what you have learned through the pages of this book.

Peter S. Jensen, MD
President and CEO
The REACH Institute

v

Preface

There are two reasons why I undertook the writing of this book. The first reason is somewhat circumstantial. More than 25 years ago, I participated in the development of a clinic called "The Center for Attention Deficit Disorders," and during the intervening years, we assessed, diagnosed, treated, and followed several thousand children with ADHD and related, and often coexistent, mental health conditions.

It was an amazing learning environment that, in addition to the diagnostic and medication management, provided other multimodality treatment necessities, including parent training (e.g., advocacy, behavior management), anger management classes, social skills classes, academic assessments, tutoring and study skills training, and a summer program for educational and behavioral enhancement.

The staff included a pediatrician (me), program assistant, RNs, and pediatric nurse practitioners, with consultation and assistance from child psychiatry, child psychology, speech/language, counseling, and education. Published research from the clinic studied the financial cost to the healthcare system of a child or an adolescent with ADHD, the effectiveness of parent training classes, and the incidence of coexistent conditions accompanying the ADHD.

The last finding, i.e., the incidence of coexisting conditions in children with ADHD, such as learning disabilities, behavior disorders, anxiety, depression, and other conditions, is the second and more important reason I undertook the writing of this book.

We discovered, as never before, that the primary care clinician, in order to diagnose, adequately treat, and manage a common problem in one's practice, such as the child with ADHD, needed the ability to recognize, diagnose, and, in many instances, provide treatment for these coexistent conditions because the incidence of comorbid conditions was so high, perhaps as high as 75% in the ADHD population. Sadly, many primary care clinicians are both inadequately trained and thus lack the self-confidence, or ability, to do so. A 2013 survey by the American Academy of Pediatrics showed that 65% of practicing pediatricians felt that they lacked the necessary training to treat mental health concerns in kids, 40% felt

they lacked the ability to diagnose these problems, and >50% lacked confidence in their ability to treat them.

The need for mental health diagnosis and treatment is so great today, even in kids without ADHD, that unless primary care clinicians (particularly pediatricians, who see the bulk of children) step up and help, the job cannot possibly ever get done. The National Institute of Mental Health estimates that about 13% of children aged 8–15 years will experience a severe mental health disorder at some point in their lives, usually before age 24 years. About 50% of these cases emerge before age 14 years, e.g., as autism, ADHD, anxiety, depression, and behavior disorders. It is estimated currently that there are at least 14 million children and adolescents in the United States in need of mental health services.

This translates to an estimated 20%–30% of current outpatient pediatric visits also involve some type of psychosocial issue. With data from the CDC National Center for Health Statistics Data Brief showing 6.1 million outpatient visits for ADHD yearly (compared with 4 million a decade earlier), the need for mental health help is increasing exponentially (48% of these outpatient visits were with pediatricians, and 80% led to prescription for stimulant medications). This is just the ADHD population, not to mention all the other children and adolescents needing mental health help.

There are even more horrific statistics. About 1:13,000 adolescents commit suicide each year, many with underlying depression. What is even more sad is that in 50% of these depressed kids, their diagnosis of depression was unrecognized and not identified by their family, peers, teachers, or primary care clinician.

So our job as pediatricians and primary care clinicians is very clear. We not only have to be competent in diagnosing and treating conditions such as adolescent anxiety and depression but also have to go looking for them!

PEARL: How? By screening all teenagers yearly, particularly the "high-risk" ones, like kids with ADHD, chronic illness, physical handicap or deformity, learning disability or school failure, parental separation or divorce, death of a parent, kids being bullied, etc. The U.S. Preventive Services Task Force recently reversed a previous position to now recommend screening for depression in **all** adolescents aged 12 years and over. This was based on their new knowledge about screening tools (such as the Patient Health Questionnaire-9 and the Beck Inventory, both proven helpful screening tools), as well as new knowledge about treatments. A previous argument that "screening could be harmful to teenagers" was successfully refuted. The American Academy of Pediatrics has also made the same recommendation, to screen all adolescents yearly for depression.

So there, my fellow primary care clinicians, is the challenge. My hope is that you are not only willing to rise to the challenge but also this resource will help give you the tools and self-confidence to do so. If we don't do it, who will?

A final word regarding who might find this resource helpful. I would envision five different levels of providers for whom the information will be very useful. (1) Clinicians who are still in training and are just starting to see patients, e.g., medical students and pediatric, psychiatric, and family practice residents. (2) Clinicians who work with us as colleagues caring for these patients, who do not prescribe medications but need to know for whom and what types of medications are helpful or indicated, side effects, etc. Examples would be counselors, family therapists, psychologists, and special education personnel. (3) Practicing clinicians such as pediatricians, family practitioners, general internists who treat adolescents, and nurse practitioners provide primary care for the bulk of these patients, and for whom it is mandatory, as expressed earlier, that they become skillful and confident in diagnosing and treating the usual straightforward types of mental health issues such as anxiety and depression. (4) Colleagues who are already providing the abovementioned mental healthcare to their patients but who want to take it to a higher level, e.g., see more complex mental health issues. Examples might be those colleagues in developmental/behavioral pediatrics, or even in child psychiatry who need information about

other practical aspects of multimodality treatment. (5) Lastly, this resource will be helpful to all the faculty in pediatrics and family practice who will be depended on to teach these principles of diagnosis and treatment to the medical students and residents but do not have the skills yet themselves, let alone the ability to teach them!

Although this is a daunting process I am confident that together we can "raise the bar" on the provision of mental health services to children. So let's get to work!

Harlan R. Gephart, MD

PS: For those wishing to receive additional training in diagnosing and treating mental health issues in children and adolescents, I strongly and enthusiastically recommend the Patient-Centered Mental Health in Primary Care (PPP) program, available through The Resource for Advancing Children's Health (REACH) Institute in New York. This is a small-group hands-on 3-day course followed by 12 biweekly conference calls with 8–10 fellow participants and led by faculty pediatricians and child psychiatrists. In this program, all aspects of mental health in children are covered, including screening, diagnosis and treatment, interviewing techniques, use of community resources, and more. It is the best educational experience I have seen or been involved with over my entire career.

Access more information at www.thereachinstitute. org.

Reference: Committee on Psychosocial Aspects of Child and Family Health and Task Force on Mental Health. Policy statement—the future of pediatrics: mental health competencies for primary care. *Pediatrics* 124:410, 2009, https://doi.org/10.1542/peds.2009-1061.

Reference: Love AR, Jensen PS, et al. The basic science of behavior change and its application to pediatric providers. *Child Adolesc Psychiatr Clin N Am* 26:851–874, 2017. (A description of The REACH Institute's Patient-Centered Mental Health in Primary Care Program.)

Acknowledgments

It is always dangerous as an author of a book to write this final section, for fear of leaving out someone who contributed to its formation. I trust I will not make that error.

I decided to become a child psychiatrist in my last year of medical school after finishing an elective clinic with a mentor named **John Kenward.** Dr. Kenward was a large "gentle giant" of a man, ex-football player at Notre Dame, who was a pediatrician turned child psychiatrist. Most of us who elected his clinic made the same career choice. He encouraged me to "study some pediatrics first" as a valuable prerequisite to child psychiatry, which I planned to do. So I entered a good pediatric residency.

Unfortunately, the Vietnam War escalated when I finished my residency, and I was forced to serve 3 years in Tripoli, Libya, as a US Air Force Pediatrician. Along the way an interesting thing happened. I loved being a general pediatrician and decided to pursue that goal, with a special interest in learning and behavioral problems of childhood. I returned to the United States, took a job on the faculty of the new University of Washington Medical School, and developed a clinic for children with "minimal brain dysfunction, which is what we called ADHD in the 1960s. I worked alongside a wonderful mentor, also a pediatrician turned child psychiatrist, **Mike Rothenberg**, whose vocational calling also focused on helping pediatricians to be more aware of and capable of diagnosing and treating children and adolescents with learning and behavioral issues. He was also a very inspiring mentor.

Then I entered practice with a large Seattle HMO, and in addition to acute and well-child care, and focused greatly on the kids with learning and behavioral issues. This led to the development of a clinic, the **Center for ADD**, in 1989, discussed in the Preface, and it was there that the accumulation of knowledge and experience in diagnosing, treating, and following several thousand children with that diagnosis occurred. It was there that we also learned that the myriad of coexistent conditions seen in children and adolescents were often more challenging than ADHD itself. In the early years, it

was "learn as you go." There was not a lot of clinical research or scientific data to go on, and even the definitions and diagnostic criteria were changing along the way. It was challenging but very rewarding work.

I want and need to mention the names of the staff at the Center for ADD who worked alongside me and made it all happen: **Maureen Green** (program assistant), **Diane Mueller**, RN (who supervised all medication refills), **Lynn McGlocklin**, ARNP (nurse practitioner who helped in the evaluation and treatment of patients), and **Sandra Shubert** and **Sandy Malone-Long** (who organized and directed the anger management/social skills classes as well as the parent training classes). Without these dedicated people the clinic as well as this book would never have become a reality.

The initial encourager for writing the book was **Paul Miles**, vice president for Quality Improvement at the American Board of Pediatrics, where I first met him. Like me, Paul had been a general pediatrician in private practice in Idaho, and like me, he also had a passion for fly-fishing. On our fishing outings, he would say, "Harlan you have to write a book about all this experience." So I finally relented.

Over the years, I was able to write articles about our experiences in the clinic, what we had learned, give continued medical education (CME) programs to physicians both in the United States and abroad, and serve in a variety of other educational venues. One such venue was the National Institute for Children's Health Quality. It was there I met **Peter Jensen**, eminent authority in ADHD research, as we developed the American Academy of Pediatrics ADHD Toolkit for primary care physicians. [I mentioned in my Preface of currently being a faculty member of Peter's The REACH (Resource for Advancing Children's Health) Institute.] Peter is the other colleague, along with Paul Miles, to insist I write of my experiences and knowledge gained in the Center for ADD. Peter is the most incredible medical educator I have ever met, and he has been an unbelievable encourager in this book endeavor. (Of course, I had to teach him some fly-fishing along the way.)

So now for some other acknowledgments. First **Marty Stein**, whom I have known from editorial boards to other CME activities that we have shared. When I decided to write the book, Marty was not only encouraging but also downright enthusiastic. Marty literally read and reviewed every paragraph I wrote and offered unbiased critique, which almost always was incorporated into the final document. Coming from someone of his stature, that was a real compliment. Marty, thank you.

Julia McMillan, nationally recognized pediatric educator at Johns Hopkins, reviewed the manuscript and wrote encouraging endorsement of its possible role in physician education, particularly the continuity clinic faculty. Thanks also to other recognized authorities in pediatric education and research, e.g., **Mark Wolraich** [colleague from ADHD Toolkit, American Board of Pediatrics (ABP), and The REACH Institute], **Ruth Stein, Suzanne Reiss, and Lynn Wegner** (three colleagues from The REACH Institute). All these people wrote helpful and encouraging comments.

Along the way in my unbelievable career, I have had the privilege of meeting and working with many talented colleagues from nonclinical areas from whom I have learned much, some of which is shared in this book. One very special person is **Sandra Rief**, a nationally recognized authority in the area of teaching children with ADHD. I have had the privilege of working with her in educational venues and have witnessed her wisdom and experience firsthand. I consider her endorsement of this book a real treasure. Likewise, **Paul Kettlewell**, clinical psychologist and Director of Mental Health Services at the Geisinger Clinics.

Particular thanks go to four authors who contributed to the actual writing: **Sam Zinner**, national authority on Tourette syndrome, who cowrote the ADHD/tics chapter; **Maya Kumar**, adolescent specialist who wrote the chapter on ADHD transitioning to adulthood; **Bob Kowatch**, child and adolescent psychiatrist, who cowrote chapters with me on bipolar disorder, aggression, and psychosis; and **Mike Jellinek**, child and adolescent psychiatrist, who graciously agreed to write a chapter on developing resilience in children and adolescents with ADHD. Thanks to you all for being a part of this effort.

I would be remiss not to mention three renowned colleagues whom I met through my participation at the ABP: **Jim Stockman** (president and CEO of the ABP), **Bob Kelch** (retired vice president and dean of the Medical School, University of Michigan), and **Jon Tingelstad** (retired chair of pediatrics, East Carolina School of Medicine). All these eminent educators, now dear personal friends to my wife and me, have been unbelievably supportive of my career and particularly my passion for kids with learning and behavioral issues. Someone else included in that group is **Bruder Stapleton**, chairman of pediatrics in my department, University of Washington School of Medicine, who sometimes introduces me as "one of his heroes." Thank you Bruder. Two others in that group of esteemed colleagues, who shared not only many years of service with me in the ABP but also long careers in the trenches of daily pediatric practice, whose endorsement of the book I really treasure, are **Jim Brown** and **Tom Roe**. Thanks to all of you wonderful friends for your support.

Thanks also to the wonderful editorial group at Elsevier, Lauren Boyle, Kristi Anderson, and especially Nadhiya Sekar, who helped me finally get it all together.

Lastly, but certainly not least, is my family. My three biological children, **Julie, Jill, and Jeff**, and two by marriage, another **Julie** and **Jon**. Most of the time in the past 2 years, they greet me with "How's the book coming?" I'm glad I can finally say "it is done, and I can really retire." To which they will say, "Dad you'll never really retire." They are probably right.

Finally, to **Kathy**, my brilliant, witty, helpful, supportive, and patient wife, who encouraged me in the writing of this book as she has done for 28 years in support of all my efforts to help the kids. Kathy, I could never thank you enough.

Harlan R. Gephart, MD
Woodinville, WA, United States

About the Author

Dr. Harlan R. Gephart received his medical education at the University of Chicago Medical School and pediatric training at the University of Washington School of Medicine. His original plans to become a child psychiatrist were delayed during the Vietnam War era, when he served as a general pediatrician with the US Air Force in Libya. Upon return to the United States, he obtained further training in behavioral pediatrics and entered practice with Group Health Cooperative (now Kaiser-Permanente) where he practiced general and behavioral pediatrics for 30 plus years.

In 1989, he helped develop a clinic called The Center for Attention Deficit Disorders to centralize care for children with attention deficit hyperactivity disorder (ADHD) and its coexistent conditions. Over the next 14 years, several thousand children were assessed, diagnosed, and treated for this condition. The clinic became a national model for using a multimodality approach to this diagnosis, consisting of parent education and training, medication, and behavioral management (see author's Preface).

Dr. Gephart remained active in medical education throughout his career, both for physicians in training as well as those already in practice, through office preceptorships, CME lectures (both nationally and internationally), and medical publications. He and his colleague Laurel Leslie developed the first online ADHD CME for the AAP's (American Academy of Pediatrics) EQUIPP program. He continues to lecture to local medical and parent groups, and is currently a consultant to Australian Family Practitioners via a skype program called ECHO.

Dr. Gephart has also been involved with the American Board of Pediatrics regarding certification of members and has served in a variety of roles such as oral examiner and board member. In 2001, he served as the Chairman of the American Board of Pediatrics.

Another passion for Dr. Gephart, arising from his tour of duty in Libya, has been the unmet medical needs in underdeveloped countries around the world. Responding to this concern, he has made more than 30 trips to countries such as Kenya, Argentina, Vietnam, Morocco, the Philippines. Of note is the country of Uzbekistan, where money ($50,000) was raised to fit over 400 deaf orphaned children with hearing aids.

In 2004 Dr. Gephart received an Honorary Doctorate in Medicine from the Tashkent Pediatric Institute for his many years of educational and humanitarian work in Uzbekistan.

ENDORSEMENTS FOR ADHD COMPLEX: PRACTICING MENTAL HEALTH IN PRIMARY CARE

1) Dr. Gephart has written an authoritative narrative on precise clinical methods that primary care pediatricians (also family practice physicians and pediatric nurse practitioners) may use when working with children and families with behavioral problems seen frequently in their offices. It is written in a manner that primary care clinicians can adapt to their practice, with loads of useful information that should lead to confidence in the diagnosis and management of children with ADHD and coexisting behavioral and learning conditions.
—**Martin T. Stein, MD**, Professor of Pediatrics Emeritus, University of California, San Diego.

2) Dr. Gephart's book is well organized and inclusive of the tools necessary to provide needed mental health care for children. ADHD comorbidities and screening tools are elaborated. Medications are well discussed. Pitfalls in diagnosis and treatment are well outlined.
—**Thomas L.W. Roe, MD**, 52 years in private practice and teaching, Clinical Professor of Pediatrics, Oregon Health Science University.

3) Dr. Gephart has extensive experience in clinically managing children with mental health conditions, particularly ADHD, as well as training pediatric

residents on those issues. He is able to blend scientific knowledge with his wealth of clinical experience.
—**Mark Wolraich, MD**, Professor of Pediatrics, Oklahoma University Child Study Center.

4) This book provides very detailed and practical help for primary care physicians in their efforts to manage mental health problems more adequately. Other health-care professionals, including pediatric psychologists and counselors, are also an appropriate audience for this book.
—**Paul Kettlewell, Ph.D.**, Director of Pediatric Psychology, The Geisinger Health System.

5) This book contains comprehensive and important information for any health-care provider taking care of children and adolescents with ADHD.
—**Danette Glassy, MD**, Pediatric Practitioner, Mercer Island, Washington. Member, AAP Task Force "Addressing Early Childhood Emotional and Behavioral Problems", 2016.

6) This book provides a wonderful foundation of knowledge, concise vignettes, practical guidelines, scientific studies to validate the information, clinical pearls, and a panoply of resource information and nonproprietary assessment tools for the busy clinician.
—**Suzanne Reiss, MD**, Child and Adolescent Psychiatrist, Faculty, The REACH Institute.

7) Not only does this book provide crucial guidance for medical and mental health practitioners to follow but also the information within is of great benefit to school psychologists, school nurses, school counselors, special education teachers, and other educators. This treasure needs to be in the hands of every school's individualized educational plan (IEP) and multidisciplinary team.
—**Sandra Rief, MA**, nationally recognized educator, consultant, and author of "How to Reach and Teach ADHD Children."

8) This book is remarkably full of practical advice for practitioners. Indeed, it seems to be a Harriet Lane Handbook for managing mental health problems in children.
—**Robert Kelch, MD**, Retired VP and Dean of the Medical School, University of Michigan.

9) The use of clinical scenarios and "pearls," complete discussion and provision of diagnostic tools, and clear treatment options including use of both behavioral and medication modalities make this an ideal resource for the busy practitioner, unlike the other currently available books on the covered subjects.
—**James Brown, MD**, 35 years of experience as pediatric practitioner, Clinical Professor of Pediatrics, Upstate Medical Center, New York.

10) Dr. Gephart is a highly respected pediatrician who is an expert and very experienced in caring for children with a variety of behavioral and mental health challenges. After reviewing this book, I came away thinking what a gift it would be for general pediatric faculty members, who are tasked with developing a curriculum to enhance their resident's competence in caring for children with behavioral and mental health problems.
—**Julia A. McMillan, MD**, Professor of Pediatrics Emeritus, Johns Hopkins School of Medicine. A lead author of "Pediatric Residency Education and the Behavioral and Mental Health Crisis. A Call to Action" PEDIATRICS.

11) Dr. Gephart has written a resource-rich book that promises to enlighten clinicians, educators, and parents about the day-to-day issues of managing youth with ADHD. Using plain English and excellent clinical examples, Dr. Gephart focuses on the recognition of the impairment that accompanies ADHD. He illustrates how it can derail social, educational, and intellectual development and what tools have proven useful to treat the symptoms of ADHD and help the patient function better. The book's detailed instructions about specific rating scales and the list of resources (books, websites, and support groups) in this book are unique and welcome. The book reads well and rewards re-reading by students, parents, and teachers. It is so good that I am using ADHD Complex: Practicing Mental Health in Primary Care for training child and adolescent psychiatrists.
—**Lawrence Greenhill, MD**, Emeritus Professor of Child and Adolescent Psychiatry, Columbia University Medical Center.

12) This book by Dr. Gephart is a gift of knowledge regarding how to diagnose and manage learning, behavioral, and mental health problems seen in children with ADHD. It is a combination of current best evidence and practical wisdom gleaned from years of actual care of children with ADHD.
—**Paul Miles, MD**, 25 plus years of experience as a practicing pediatrician, VP for Quality Improvement, American Board of Pediatrics (retired).

13) This valuable textbook provides in-depth insights into children and their families with ADHD and reminds us that these children grow into adults with residual concerns. Unfortunately, the number of mental health professional available to treat children with ADHD falls far short of the demand, leaving many children without needed services. Pediatricians and other primary care clinicians must now fill this behavioral health-care gap. Dr. Gephart is a tremendous role model for how pediatricians can provide outstanding care for children with ADHD. He offers, through this highly informative text, tools for pediatricians, allied health providers, and trainees to both understand the spectrum of ADHD and treat the many comorbidities and mental health associations. Through clinical pearls and case vignettes, the reader gains an outstanding perspective of the impact of ADHD on patients and family and how to overcome these challenges. I congratulate Dr. Gephart for this outstanding contribution to the care of children and consider it a new classic resource for the problem of ADHD.
—**F. Bruder Stapleton, MD**, Professor of Pediatrics and Associate Dean, University of Washington School of Medicine.

Contents

CHAPTER 1

Rating Scales, Questionnaires, and Behavior Checklists

First some comments about using screening tools, rating scales, behavioral checklists, etc. THEY ARE NOT DIAGNOSTIC OF ANY SPECIFIC CONDITION. They are used as preliminary instruments to gather information that may indicate a potential diagnosis or diagnoses that then need to be confirmed by obtaining more information, perhaps by using a more specific tool for a specific condition, by collecting more data, e.g., school information, by conducting a one-on-one interview with the patient, etc.

In a clinical setting, e.g., a yearly physical examination (PE) for an adolescent, one might use a behavioral checklist, such as the Guidelines for Adolescent Preventive Services (GAPS), that has a lot of questions regarding safety, high-risk behavior, school and social well-being, etc., which then help the clinician to focus on areas where interventions seem indicated.

If mental health concerns are suggested, then one might follow up with another tool mentioned later, the Pediatric Symptom Checklist (PSC). This tool further focuses on emotional and attentional concerns, in the areas of internalizing (anxiety, depression) feelings, externalizing (behavioral) issues, and attention (school progress). The results might then serve as a prompt to further narrow down the concerns by using more specific tools described later: Screen for Child Anxiety Disorders (SCARED, anxiety), Patient Health Questionnaire (PHQ)-9 (depression), and Vanderbilt (academic).

These tools take only a few minutes to complete, can be scored easily by the office staff, and can be optimally obtained prior to the appointment, or while in the waiting room prior to being seen by the clinician. They are immense TIMESAVERS in the evaluation process, and although not totally diagnostic in themselves, they contribute greatly to the diagnostic process.

Obviously if the stated reason for the appointment is a specific issue, such as rule out (R/O) depression or R/O ADHD, then the clinician might choose to go directly to the specific screening tool, along with appropriate history and physical examination.

PEARL: Rating scales are by and large billable, e.g., Vanderbilt, SCARED, PHQ-9, PSC. Behavior checklists are usually considered to be extensions of the history component of the evaluation and are not billable, e.g., Modified Overt Aggression Scale (MOAS), GAPS.

PEARL: Most pediatricians in practice are quite familiar and adept at using the Vanderbilt questionnaires for assessing ADHD. This chapter will describe other screening tools that, although not completely diagnostic of certain mental health conditions such as anxiety and depression, are very important to use in the assessment of such conditions. So if the clinician is going to diagnose and/or treat complex ADHD, which basically means the assessment for all the potential coexistent conditions, such as anxiety, depression, aggression, and possible bipolar disorder, he or she must become knowledgeable about and must be able to use other rating scales in addition to the Vanderbilt or Connor scale (that is what this book is all about.). These tools are described fully in this chapter and are also essentially all available free online, unless noted otherwise.

RATING SCALES AND BEHAVIORAL CHECKLISTS

A. Behavioral checklists

1). GAPS
   - Free, available through the American Medical Association (GAPS-HSR form)
   - A questionnaire, not a "rating scale" per se
   - For adolescents, aged 11—21 years
     - Contains 72 questions for teens regarding risk behaviors such as drinking, smoking, sex, drugs, and car safety (based on the four most frequent causes of death in teens—motor vehicle accidents, other accidents, suicide, and homicide)
     - Used by the clinician for the "Identification and Treatment of Risk Behaviors"

- Has two forms: younger adolescent and older adolescent
- Can be completed easily by an adolescent within a few minutes in the waiting room prior to the appointment
- Mnemonics are useful to categorize discussion topics, e.g., SAFE TEENS

S	Sexuality	T	Toxins, tobacco, accidents, abuse
A	Anxiety	E	Environment (school, home)
F	Firearms, homicide	E	Exercise
E	Suicide, depression	N	Nutrition
		S	Shots (immunizations, school)

- Should be used at least annually during annual PE, sports PE, or any other visit

2). **PSC-17**
- New version (older version had 35 questions)
- Parent version (for children/adolescents aged 4−16 years)
- Youth version (ages 11−18 years)
- Useful for screening for psychosocial issues in primary care
- Although it is scored, it is not a definitive diagnostic tool
- Rather, it "suggests areas that need more evaluation"
- Measures three domains
  Externalizing
  Internalizing
  Attention
- Available free online, www.massgeneral.org/psychiatry/services/psc_forms.aspx
- Most useful in a general pediatric setting as a preliminary tool if a concern arises regarding mood disorder, behavioral problems, or ADHD issues
- If suggestive of concerns in those areas follow up with more specific rating scales (e.g., Vanderbilt, SCARED, PHQ-9) as well as a one-on-one interview (recommended)

B. **Broadband rating scales**

Broadband rating scales are lengthy questionnaires (e.g., 100 or more questions) that score responses/information regarding several domains of the child's life. On the positive side, they screen for many problems/concerns. On the negative side, they obviously screen more superficially and thus should never be used as a definitive diagnostic tool.

Nonetheless, they can be very helpful as an initial screen. Two widely used broadband rating scales are discussed in the following. They are both proprietary and, therefore, not available for free online like other screening tools.

1) **Child Behavior Checklist**
- Also called the "Achenbach" after its developer; proprietary, not free
- Contains about 120 questions and covers ages 6−13 years
- Has parent, teacher, and child forms
- Also has a preschool form, for ages 18 months to 5 years
- Covers/screens for symptoms suggesting ADHD, oppositional defiant disorder, conduct disorder, depression, anxiety, phobias, and others
- Also develops scores for aggressive behavior and internalizing and externalizing problems
- Scores are reported as normal, borderline, or the clinical behavior
- Used most often by clinical psychologists and school psychologists, not often by clinicians, but we need to be familiar with it because it will be seen in school reports
- Any concerns that are noted should be followed up by more specific screening and interviews to make a definitive diagnosis

2). **Behavior Assessment System for Children (Edition 2)**
- Proprietary, not free
- Used commonly by school and clinical psychologists, child psychiatrists
- Has teacher [teacher rating scale (TRS)], parent [parent rating scale (PRS)], and child/self [self-rating scale (SRS)] versions
- Covers ages from 2 to 25 years
- Used commonly prior to a clinical interview to focus on specific areas
- Scores conditions such as hyperactivity, aggression, atypicality, withdrawal, and attention
- Schools seem to use this instrument, as very often screening is being done for ADHD
- Disadvantage: The self-report does not screen for specific emotional disorders, substance abuse, and alcohol abuse

- Any concerns that surface on this screening tool should be followed up by more specific screening tools as well as by a clinical interview
- Available at www.BASC-2Summary-basc-2.szopkiw.com

C. **Specific rating scales**

Following are the specific rating scales designed to screen for and quantitate specific diagnoses or concerns, e.g., ADHD, anxiety, depression, aggression, and mania.

However, it should be reiterated that RATING SCALES DO NOT MAKE A DEFINITIVE DIAGNOSIS.

They suggest specific diagnoses that must be confirmed by more information, clinical interviews, etc.

1). **Vanderbilt ADHD Diagnostic Rating Scales**
   - Free; available online at https://soonersuccess.ouhsc.edu/
   - Measures ADHD cardinal symptoms (inattention, hyperactivity, and impulsivity)
   - Has parent and teacher versions
   - Includes questions to measure "functional impairment" as well (at school, home, etc.)
   - Parent version screens (briefly) for oppositional defiant disorder, conduct disorder, anxiety, and depression
   - Teacher version also screens for mood disorders and anxiety symptoms, as well as behavioral issues
   - Follow-up Vanderbilt forms (briefer) are helpful for monitoring the control of ADHD core symptoms as well as impairment, even though they do not screen for coexisting conditions but only for the ADHD symptoms and impairment. For this reason, some clinicians continue to use the larger Vanderbilt questionnaire as a follow-up form as well.

PEARL: Based on a study from Cincinnati the Vanderbilt is also a good screening tool for learning disabilities. Langberg JM, Vaughn AJ, Brinkman WB, Froehlich T, and Epstein JN. Learning Disorders: Clinical Utility of the Vanderbilt ADHD Rating Scale for Ruling Out Comorbid Learning Disabilities. *Pediatrics* 126(5):e1033–8, 2010.

2). **PHQ-9 (modified for teens): Depression**
   - Available free online (American Academy of Pediatrics (AAP): www.brightfutures.org)
   - Useful for the diagnosis of depression as well as for monitoring symptoms over time

- Not diagnostic in itself—needs to be confirmed with clinical symptoms and interviews
- Questions are all self-reported, and hence the need to be verified by clinical interviews and observation
- Has excellent validity
  Sensitivity, 88%
  Specificity, 88%
- The scores below indicate the likelihood of a diagnosis of Major Depression
  0–4, No evidence
  5–9, Minimal evidence
  10–14, Minor depression
  15–19, Moderately severe depression
  >20, Severe depression

3). **SCARED**
   - Available free online, www.pediatricbipolar.pitt.edu or www.dbp2doc.org
   - Has child and parent versions
   - Has good reliability and validity
   - Sensitive to treatment response (therefore excellent for serial monitoring)
   - Used for children aged 8–18 years
   - Can be scored by hand or automatically
   - Also measures subtypes of anxiety, e.g., separation, social phobia, panic, school phobia
   - Most experts feel the subtypes overlap too much in children, or merge with time, so that discrimination of subtypes is not that valid or helpful

4). **MOAS**
   - Available free online, www.cappcny.org/home/documents
   - Rates four types of aggressive behavior: verbal, property, autoaggression (to self), and physical
   - Used by clinicians to assess degree/type of aggressive behavior
   - Also used by clinicians to track/monitor aggressive behavior, e.g., monitor response to treatment
   - Has good reliability and validity

5). **The Young Mania Rating Scale (Dr. Young was the developer)**
   - Has parent and teacher forms
   - 11-Item, multiple-choice questionnaire
   - Helpful in diagnosis of bipolar disorder in children/adolescents but has high false-positive rate
   - High scores suggest "risk" of bipolar disorder

Scores 0–60
>13 suggests "potential mania"
>21 suggests "probable mania"
- Can also be used to monitor "response to management"
- Available free online

6). **The Modified Nisonger Child Behavior Rating Form (NCBRF)**
- Originally designed for assessing behavior in children with intellectual disability, autism, etc.
- Now, new edition, NCBRF–TIQ is available for assessing behavior in children/adolescents with "typical development"
- Assesses for conduct problems, oppositional, hyperactive, inattentive, withdrawn, dysphoric, and overly sensitive
- Has teacher and parent versions
- For ages 3–16 years
- More suitable to follow behavior serially, e.g., response to interventions, rather than as a diagnostic tool
- Available free
  Contact: The Nisonger Center
  Dr. Aman
  Ohio State University
  Columbus, OH 43210-1296, United States
  Aman.l@osu.edu

7). **CRAFFT (substance abuse)**
- For adolescents aged <21 years
- Often used along with the GAPS questionnaire
- Has six questions; screens for high-risk drug and alcohol usage/abuse
- Short and effective tool
- Questions are asked by clinician using exact wording in the questionnaire
  C. Have you ever ridden in a CAR driven by someone, including yourself, who was "high" or had been using alcohol or drugs?
  R. Do you ever use alcohol or drugs to RELAX, feel better about yourself, or fit in?
  A. Do you ever use alcohol/drugs while you are by yourself ALONE?
  F. Do you ever FORGET things you did while using alcohol or drugs?
  F. Do your family or FRIENDS ever tell you that you should cut down on your drinking or drug use?

T. Have you gotten into TROUBLE while you were using alcohol or drugs?
- Free; available at AAP www.brightfutures.org and ceasar@childrens.harvard.edu

8). **Adult ADHD Self-Report Scale**
- 18-Question self-report
- Has two parts
  A. Inattentive traits
  B. Hyperactive/impulsive traits
- Score
  0–16, ADHD unlikely
  17–23, ADHD likely
  24 or more, ADHD highly likely
- Also assesses presence of functional impairment (e.g., home life, job, social)
- Needs to be correlated with patient's history, PE, and evidence of other mental health issues (e.g., anxiety, depression) that may "mimic" ADHD or be a coexisting problem

PEARL: This questionnaire can be used to explore possible ADHD in a parent of the child/adolescent patient with ADHD (statistically ~50% of parents of children with ADHD had/have ADHD). It would be very helpful to diagnose and treat him/her, if needed.

PEARL: The ADHD remaining symptom traits may be subthreshold, but impairment and fallout from earlier ADHD might be major (anxiety/depression, substance abuse, etc.)
- Available free at https://med.nyu.edu/psych/adhd-self-assessment-tools-and-information

9). **Adolescent ADHD self-report (Ages 12–18 Years)**: Available online (not free), www.drthomasebrown.com/assessment-tools.

10). **Edinburgh Postnatal Depression Scale:** Use this tool to screen for postnatal depression. Available free online at www.brightfutures.org.

Reference for website screening tool and rating scale: http://www.heardalliance.org/wp-content/uploads/2011/04/Mental-Health-Assessment.pdf

Following is a questionnaire for parents with academic and/or behavioral concerns about their child. Used by permission from Allegro Pediatrics, Bellevue, WA, United States. (May be reprinted for personal clinical use as long as the name of the clinic [Allegro Pediatrics, Bellevue, WA, United States] and the name of the author [Harlan R. Gephart, MD] are acknowledged.)

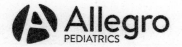

Questionnaire for Parents with
Academic and/or Behavioral Concerns about their Child
Developed in collaboration with the expertise and experience of Harlan Gephart, MD

This form must be completed before your next visit to help your physician with the evaluation.

Name of Child: _____ Birth Date: _____

Names of Parent(s): _____

Contact Phone Number(s): _____

School Name: _____ District: _____ Grade: _____

Name of Teacher(s): _____

Contact Phone Number for Teacher(s): _____

Briefly list academic and behavioral concerns about your child, starting with the most concerning:

1. _____

2. _____

3. _____

4. _____

5. _____

Please complete this questionnaire and the Vanderbilt Assessment Scales (with one completed by the teacher) about your child as best as possible. Thank you for your time and help with this important part of the evaluation.

E.MIC.F5.072815b.0315c

For Office Use
Provider's Initials _____
Date Reviewed _____

Circle **Yes** or **No** to the following questions.

Pregnancy, delivery, and early infancy
1. Where was your baby born? _____
    a. Birth weight ___lb ___oz
2. More active in utero than siblings? Yes / No
3. Did you smoke during pregnancy? Yes / No
4. Did you drink alcohol during pregnancy? Yes / No
5. Was the delivery "difficult"? Yes / No
6. Was the delivery a C-section? Yes / No
7. Did your baby need oxygen? Yes / No
8. Baby need vigorous resuscitation? Yes / No
9. Baby in hospital after Mom discharged? Yes / No

General health and daily life
10. Is your child a "daredevil" or risk taker? Yes / No
11. Has many accidents/injuries? Yes / No
12. Has your child ever ingested a poison? Yes / No
13. Has your child ever had a seizure? Yes / No
14. Head injury with loss of consciousness? Yes / No
15. Serious illness or hospitalization? Yes / No
16. Any history of physical or sexual abuse? Yes / No
17. Does your child have a sleep problem? Yes / No
    a. Difficulty falling asleep? Yes / No
    b. Restless sleep? Yes / No
    c. Hard to awaken? Yes / No
18. Problems getting ready for school? Yes / No
    a. Needs reminders? Yes / No
    b. Gets distracted? Yes / No
    c. Would be late unless prodded? Yes / No
    d. Forgets usual order of routine? Yes / No
19. Problems handling changes of schedule? Yes / No
20. Problems with transitions? Yes / No
    a. Warnings and preparation help? Yes / No

Activity Level
21. Is your child "hyperactive"? Yes / No
22. Is your child "fidgety and wiggly"? Yes / No
23. Have trouble sitting through meals? Yes / No
24. Avoid restaurants because of your child? Yes / No
25. Is shopping more difficult for this child? Yes / No
26. Do you avoid taking your child shopping? Yes / No
27. Cannot sit quietly and watch TV? Yes / No
28. Often doing something else at same time? Yes / No
29. Does your child talk excessively? Yes / No
30. Is this annoying at times? Yes / No
31. Make strange/unusual noises during play? Yes / No
32. Does your child have a tic? Yes / No

Family History
33. Is there any Family History on either side of:
    a. Cardiac Problems? Yes / No
    b. Learning Problems/Disorders? Yes / No
    c. Attention deficit disorder? Yes / No
    d. Tics or Tourette Disorder? Yes / No
    e. Depression? Yes / No
    f. Anxiety Disorder? Yes / No
    g. Bipolar Disorder? Yes / No
    h. Substance Abuse or Alcoholism? Yes / No
    i. Adolescent Problems? Yes / No
    j. School Drop-out? Yes / No
    k. Being Held Back in School? Yes / No
    l. Trouble with the Law? Yes / No

Early Development
34. Abnormal early development landmarks? Yes / No
    a. Late sitting up (after 8 months)? Yes / No
    b. Late walking (after 15 months)? Yes / No
    c. Late single words (after 18 mo)? Yes / No
    d. Late small phrases (after 2 yrs)? Yes / No
    e. Late sentences (after 3 years)? Yes / No
35. Late in toilet training? Yes / No
36. Late in staying dry at night? Yes / No
37. Have accidents with stool? Yes / No

Motor Coordination
38. Problems in large motor coordination? Yes / No
    a. Problems throwing/catching ball? Yes / No
    b. Problems running/jumping? Yes / No
    c. Problems riding a bicycle? Yes / No
39. Problems with fine motor coordination? Yes / No
    a. Problems with tying shoes? Yes / No
    b. Problems coloring in the lines? Yes / No
    c. Problems with handwriting? Yes / No
    d. Problems with using scissors? Yes / No
40. Does your child dislike team sports? Yes / No
41. Attention problems in games/practice? Yes / No
42. Difficult to read his/her handwriting? Yes / No
43. If yes, would writing more slowly help? Yes / No

Attentional and Organizational Abilities
44. Inattentive during non-school activities? Yes / No
    a. Inattentive during chores? Yes / No
    b. Inattentive dressing/bedtime? Yes / No
45. Difficulty with multiple instruction? Yes / No
46. Distracted easily during homework? Yes / No
    a. Procrastinates? Yes / No
    b. Gets up and down? Yes / No
    c. Needs help 1-on-1 to stay on task? Yes / No
    d. Takes very long to finish work? Yes / No
47. Problems with short-term memory? Yes / No
    a. Loses and misplaces things? Yes / No
    b. Forgets things at school? Yes / No
    c. Forgets to turn in homework? Yes / No
    d. Loses or misplaces homework? Yes / No

    e. Problems remembering dates?   Yes / No
48. Difficulty with school projects?   Yes / No
    a. Difficulty making an outline?   Yes / No
    b. Difficulty breaking into steps?   Yes / No
    c. Easily overwhelmed by projects?   Yes / No
    d. 1-on-1 helps dramatically?   Yes / No
49. Does your child daydream a lot?   Yes / No
50. Does "space cadet" describe your child?   Yes / No

Impulsivity
51. Fascinated by matches, setting fires?   Yes / No
52. Make impulsive statements?   Yes / No
    a. Problems with interrupting?   Yes / No
    b. Problems with blurting out?   Yes / No
53. Any inappropriate behaviors?   Yes / No
    a. Rude or obnoxious?   Yes / No
    b. Bossy or controlling?   Yes / No
    c. Competitive or need to win?   Yes / No
    d. Ignores or disobeys rules?   Yes / No
    e. "In your face"?   Yes / No
    f. Inappropriate touching?   Yes / No
    g. Doesn't read social cues?   Yes / No
    h. Doesn't learn from experience?   Yes / No
    i. Repeats same mistakes?   Yes / No
54. Does your child have anger problems?   Yes / No
    a. Hitting or fighting?   Yes / No
    b. Breaking or throwing objects?   Yes / No
    c. Destroying property?   Yes / No
55. Any problems with friendships?   Yes / No
    a. Few or no friends?   Yes / No
    b. Rare party invitations/playdates?   Yes / No
    c. Prefers younger/older children?   Yes / No
    d. Immature compared to peers?   Yes / No
    e. Makes friends but loses them?   Yes / No

Other Associated Behaviors
56. Does your child have poor self-esteem?   Yes / No
    a. Self-derogatory statements?   Yes / No
    b. Acts sad or depressed?   Yes / No
    c. Withdraws?   Yes / No
    d. Verbalizes death wish/statement?   Yes / No
57. Does your child ever appear anxious?   Yes / No
    a. Panic attacks?   Yes / No
    b. Hyperventilation?   Yes / No
    c. Specific fears or phobias?   Yes / No
58. Any obsessive-compulsive behavior?   Yes / No
59. Does your child lie?   Yes / No
    a. Refuses to admit responsibility?   Yes / No
    b. Makes up untrue stories?   Yes / No
60. Does your child steal?   Yes / No
    a. Shoplift?   Yes / No
    b. Money from home, others' toys?   Yes / No

61. Ever abused any substance?   Yes / No
    a. Cigarettes?   Yes / No
    b. Alcohol?   Yes / No
    c. Marijuana?   Yes / No
    d. Other illicit drugs?   Yes / No
62. Any association with a gang?   Yes / No
63. Is your child sexually active?   Yes / No
64. Problems with obedience/compliance?   Yes / No
    a. Argumentative?   Yes / No
    b. Oppositional or Defiant?   Yes / No
    c. Blames others?   Yes / No
    d. Refuses to accept responsibility?   Yes / No
65. What disciplinary techniques are helpful?
    a. Time-outs?   Yes / No
    b. Consequence systems?   Yes / No
    c. Reward systems?   Yes / No
    d. Restriction of privileges?   Yes / No
    e. Nothing works?   Yes / No
66. been involved in antisocial behavior?   Yes / No
    a. Setting fires?   Yes / No
    b. Breaking and entering?   Yes / No
    c. Physical violence with weapon?   Yes / No
    d. Cruelty to animals or peers?   Yes / No
67. Contact with police/juvenile authorities?   Yes / No
68. Currently involved with a counselor?   Yes / No
69. If yes, contact info. _____

Academic Concerns
70. Is your child below grade level? How much?
    a. Reading? _____ Yes / No
    b. Math? _____ Yes / No
    c. Writing? _____ Yes / No
71. Teacher raise concerns about progress?   Yes / No
72. If yes, at what grade level and what concerns in
    a. Academics? _____
    b. Behavior? _____
73. School testing for learning disabilities?   Yes / No
74. Any private learning evaluations?   Yes / No
75. Any private tutoring?   Yes / No
76. What contributes to academic difficulties?
    a. Not paying attention in class?   Yes / No
    b. Not finishing all the homework?   Yes / No
    c. Homework lost, late, forgotten?   Yes / No
    d. Doesn't study for tests?   Yes / No
    e. Hurried, careless, not proofread?   Yes / No
    f. Doesn't understand material?   Yes / No
77. Addendum:
    • One or two parents?_____
    • Sibling relationships OK?   Yes / No
    • Blended family?   Yes / No
    • Foster child?   Yes / No
    • Separation/Divorce?   Yes / No
    • Describe Living/Sleeping Arrangements_____
    • Describe Custody Rules(joint/sole etc.)_____

CHAPTER 2

Learning Problems in Children and Adolescents

WHAT IS A SPECIFIC LEARNING DISORDER?

Case Vignette: Rachel is an 8-year-old third grader. Parents bring her in because the teacher has noted that she is inattentive and distractible, but not hyperactive. These symptoms had been noted since first grade, and now the concern was heightened because she was falling behind academically. For example, recent preliminary testing by the teacher showed 6–12 months delay in reading skills.

Workup in the clinic confirmed that Rachel met criteria for ADHD, inattentive type. Concern was raised that a subtle learning disorder might be a possibility as well. She was begun on ADHD medication, with marked improvement in her ADHD symptoms, e.g., better attention span, and concentration. However, after 3 months of treatment, the teacher reported "something wasn't right yet." "She seems smart enough and attentive to do better." Referral for an individualized educational plan (IEP) testing was done that revealed "normal IQ" but the presence of a subtle learning disorder in reading.

Perhaps the first question to ask is, "Why does a primary care clinician need to know what a specific learning disorder is? Isn't that the role of the school system?"

To be sure, the school bears the major responsibility for education of the child/adolescent. However, if the primary care clinician is to serve as the overseer of the child/adolescent's well-being in many areas, including growth and development, social and peer relations, family interactions, chronic illness or disabilities, he or she needs to know how school success and the learning process can be negatively impacted by medical issues.

For example, the primary care clinician needs to know

1). the risk factors for having a learning problem,
2). the association between certain medical and/or genetic conditions and learning problems,
3). the clues in the child's medical or developmental history that would alert one of a concern of possible learning issues.

All this will be summarized in greater detail in the following. So let us go back to the initial question: "What is a specific learning disorder?"

A. Specific learning disorder (SLD) has replaced previous terms such as learning problem and learning disability. SLD is now presumed to be a neurodevelopmental disorder, which is the term used when a child has impaired ability to process information, presumably on a genetic or neurologic basis and independent of intelligence or cognitive ability.
  1). Types of SLD (problem areas)
    • reading aloud
    • understanding what is read
    • spelling
    • writing
    • math calculations
    • math reasoning
  2). The problems may be subtle; they may be apparent early in school years, or later.
  3). The problems result in functioning markedly below expectations for age and/or cognitive ability.
  4). The problems are impairing to some areas of life (school, job, etc.).
B. Additional information regarding SLD
  1). There are no apparent biological markers of SLD.
  2). Neuroimaging is not helpful in diagnosis.
  3). It is often preceded by delay in language skills.
  4). It occurs unrelated to a person's level of cognitive ability or IQ.
  5). It often results in secondary mental health concerns presumably due to school failure.
C. Epidemiology of SLD
  1). About 12%–15% occurrence rate in general population

2). Perhaps 25% or so occurrence in children with ADHD

3). More common in males, 2:1 or so

4). Less frequent in nonalphabet languages, e.g., Chinese

5). SLD may cause symptoms similar to ADHD (inattention, distractibility) and may be either incorrectly diagnosed as ADHD or a missed coexistent diagnosis in a child with ADHD

PEARL: If you have a child with SLD rule out ADHD, and vice versa, as the coexistent problem.

D. Frequent precursors and/or risk factors

1). Prematurity or low birth weight, small for gestational age

2). Genetics (5%–10% higher incidence in first-degree relatives)

3). Speech delay, or language disorder

4). Delay in "phonologic awareness" (differentiating sounds)

- Associated with reading and writing problems, e.g., dyslexia

PEARL: Hence, kindergarteners and first graders are tested as a predictor for potential issues later on (poor "phonologic awareness" is a risk factor or "predictor" of reading disorders).

5) ADHD (per comments mentioned earlier)

E. Prognosis of having an SLD

1). Lower academic attainment (e.g., less likely to go to college)

2). Greater likelihood of dropping out of high school

3). Increase in mental health issues, e.g., depression

4). Increase in unemployment or underemployment

5). Lower income as an adult

F. Coexistent conditions often seen with SLD

1). ADHD

2). Mental conditions: anxiety, depression, and bipolar disorder

3). Autism

4). Communication disorder

5). Behavior disorders (oppositional defiant disorder, conduct disorder)

G. Clues to possible learning disorders

1). Family history of dyslexia or learning disorder

2). Delayed language development

3). Letter/number reversal after 7 years of age

4). Difficulty with reading, writing, or math despite 1:1 adult supervision

5). Congenital malformations (e.g., heart, orthopedic anomalies)

6). Medical syndromes (e.g., Williams syndrome, Turner syndrome, etc.)/genetic disorders

7). Academic delays of >6 months

8). Academic underachievement despite appropriate ADHD treatment

9). Adolescent dislike for school or poor success in school

All the abovementioned are **PEARL**.

H. Differential diagnosis of SLD (not a complete list)

1). Lower IQ, e.g., 70

2). Sensory disorders (auditory, visual)

3). Neurologic disorders (e.g., near drowning, traumatic brain injury, seizures)

4). Neurodegenerative conditions

5). ADHD

I. Treatment of SLD: For example, special education, tutoring, other school accommodations will be discussed later.

WHAT IS THE INDIVIDUALS WITH DISABILITIES EDUCATION ACT?

Questions

1). Who is helped by this federal law?

2). What services does it offer?

3). How does a patient/parent access these services?

A. History

The Individuals with Disabilities Education Act (IDEA) is the current version of the original federal law called "Education for all Handicapped Children Law" passed by Congress in 1975. This law mandates that all children with disabilities receive free and appropriate public education (FAPE). The federal government provides money yearly to all the states to develop and provide special education programs (regular education is financed and provided by each state, not the federal government).

Periodically the law, now known as IDEA, gets reauthorized (funded) by Congress and, in the process, changes are sometimes made to the law. The current revision was authorized in 2004 and included some major changes, which will be discussed in the following.

B. The main components of the IDEA 2004 Federal law required the following from the states:

1). FAPE for each child/adolescent.

2). Parents to be involved with the schools as equal partners in the decision-making process of their child.

3). The evaluations and assessments would be nondiscriminatory.

4). Each child would receive an IEP that took into account his/her needs, strengths, parents' wishes, results of testing, etc.

5). The education would be provided in the least restrictive environment, e.g., the child will not be removed from a regular classroom to a special education room if needs could be met in a regular classroom.

6). Right for parents to due process.

C. Major changes to IDEA in the 2004 reauthorization (from previous versions of the law)

1). Elimination of the "severe discrepancy" concept. Prior to 2004, to be accepted into special education, the student needed a "severe discrepancy" between academic potential, as measured by IQ testing, and current performance. This was usually about a 2-year delay. So, if the child did not qualify, he/she received no services or accommodations and, as expected, eventually fell behind enough academically to qualify (this was called the "wait-to-fail" rule). Many children, as a result, did not receive special education until their falling behind had worsened.

IDEA 2004 eliminated "severe discrepancy" as a requirement for providing services and allowed other factors to be used in the evaluation and in the decision process.

2). It gave the schools a new tool, i.e., "response to intervention (RTI)," as a new factor to be used in the determination of need (and qualification) for special education services.

D. What is RTI? (summarized)

1). Definition: A process (included in IDEA 2004) that provides evidence-based instruction and a tiered continuum of intervention to children who struggle to learn, hopefully in the general education program, thus reducing the need for special education.

2). Components of RTI

- screening program in early school years to identify "at-risk" students and to circumvent the "wait-to-fail" concept,
- all scientifically proven educational techniques,
- multiple levels of interventions,
- constant monitoring of the student's progress,
- parental involvement in decisions regarding the student's accommodations,
- all instructions by highly qualified persons.

3). Benefits of RTI

- increases success rate in general education, reducing referrals to and the need for special education services,
- increases quality of instruction in general classrooms,
- reduces time and waiting list for students to get help,
- eliminates some unnecessary testing for the special education evaluation process.

4). Potential disadvantages of RTI for students with learning disorders

- does not give schools specific instructions on how to evaluate children who do not respond to RTI,
- not every school has the highly trained personnel to provide RTI,
- there is no specification in the law regarding the length of time the student must be in RTI before receiving a special education evaluation.

E. IDEA 2004: For whom and how it is applied

1). Applies to children with "disabilities" and specifies their educational rights

2). There are 13 separate disability categories:

- specific learning disability
- auditory disability
- visual disability
- orthopedic disability
- neurologic disability
- emotional disability
- developmental disability
- autism
- behavioral disability
- other health impairment (OHI)
- traumatic brain injury
- speech/language disability
- intellectual disability

3). What is OHI?

- Definition: The health problem causes "limited strength, vitality, or alertness" at school, thus requiring special education.
- Examples: Diabetes, Tourette syndrome, asthma, congenital heart problems, etc.

PEARL: Includes ADHD.

- OHI requirements vary by states, e.g., some require physician signatures, some do not.
- The school will gather information and do an evaluation to see if the child meets OHI requirements.

4). Under IDEA, all students in special education must have an IEP

5). IEP features (partial list)
- Tailored to each child's specific needs
- Developed by school's multidisciplinary team, which consists of personnel such as regular education teacher, special education teacher, school principal, counselor, school psychologist, and speech and language pathologist, etc.
- Helps in forming all educational decisions
- Annual review of progress
- Interventions/accommodations at no cost to parents
- Parents help formulate the IEP

PEARL: Eligibility for special education is not based on academic failure only.

6). IDEA and ADHD
   a) ADHD may qualify for special education if meeting the criteria in three different categories:
- specific learning disability (SLD)
- OHI

      PEARL: Most common way to qualify is OHI.
- emotional disturbance

   b) All concerns regarding the child (learning, emotional, behavioral, executive function, etc.) should be addressed by the IEP.

7). Other services provided by IDEA 2004 (this is a partial list):
- speech/language services,
- occupational and/or physical therapy,
- transportation,
- psychological services,
- school health services.

8). Ways to obtain IDEA services (this is a partial list):
- school person or parent initiate referral,
- school reviews the child's functioning and may (or may not) determine evaluation is indicated,
- parents must give consent for testing,
- assessment must include the specific area of concern,
- evaluation must be done by qualified personnel,
- the evaluation must be done in the language deemed most accurate for the child.
- a school has 60 calendar days to complete the evaluation,
- if the school refuses to do an evaluation then parents may request a "due process hearing,"

- IEPs are reviewed annually
- complete reevaluation (regarding need for continuing services) is done every 3 years unless parents and the school agree it is not necessary.

PEARL: Children in private schools are eligible for testing (and some accommodations) at the public school in their neighborhood (parents are obligated to provide transportation.).

Reference: Lipkin P, et al. The Individuals with Disabilities Education Act (IDEA) for children with special educational needs. *Pediatrics.* 2015;136:e1650–e1662.

IEP TESTING

Case Vignette: Peter is a 14-year-old boy brought to you because he ran away from home. When asked by you alone how that occurred, he stated that he "hated school."

Peter had previously been diagnosed with ADHD, combined type, in elementary school and was given ADHD medication. Subsequently, his grades improved because of his improved focus and work completion. Now his previous failing grades were "average."

When you interviewed Peter, you were amazed at how intelligent he seemed, for someone getting only "average grades," e.g., he named all the planets and several star constellations and said he wanted to be an astronomer or physicist. When asked why he hated school, he said that it was "hard for him."

IEP testing was arranged and it revealed that Peter's IQ was 140, but he suffered from a severe specific learning disability that, along with his ADHD, made school not only boring but also extremely difficult for him.

What tests must be done? A school-based psychoeducational assessment as part of the evaluation for special education eligibility may involve a number of tests administered by the school psychologist and other qualified specialists of the IEP team. Some of these tests are discussed in the following.

1). Cognitive (IQ) testing (measures level of intelligence)
- Has to be 1:1 testing
- Some parts are timed, some are untimed
- Two tests are "gold standard" (except in children with language impairment)
Wechsler Intelligence Scale for Children (WISC-V), which is basically the test universally done
Stanford-Binet test

2). Achievement (measures the level of current performance in reading, writing, and mathematics)
- Tests used for measuring achievement must be "nationally normed," i.e., proven to be accurate and reliable across population groups, etc.
- Examples:
  Woodcock-Johnson (WJ IV) test
    measures reading, writing, and mathematics
  Wechsler Individual Achievement Test (WIAT IV)
    measures reading, writing, and mathematics
  Key Math (rarely used any more)
    measures mathematics
  Wide-Range Achievement Test (WRAT)
    measures several academic skills
    older test, less accurate, but easier to perform
    (Actually, the WRAT is really only a "screening test" and is not part of the current officially recognized IEP tests but may occasionally be used or mentioned by the tester in the report.) Curriculum-based assessment and other informal measures may also be included.

3). Processing tests (of auditory and visual functioning, fine and gross motor functioning, etc.)
- These tests are often optional, though some are usually included in the IEP testing, and are usually done by the occupational and physical therapists and speech/language pathologists.

4). Executive functioning
- Behavior Rating Inventory of Executive Function (BRIEF) questionnaire
- Has adult and child versions
- Child versions
  BRIEF (5–18 years)
  BRIEF P (Preschool, 2–6 years)
  BRIEF SR (Self-Report, 8–18 years)
- Parents and teachers complete BRIEF
- Parents or day care completes BRIEF P
- Adolescent completes BRIEF SR
- Proprietary, not available for free
- Measures skills such as planning, organizing, monitoring, working memory, and adaptability to changes

PEARL: Most kids, adolescents, and adults (though not all) with ADHD have major problems with executive functioning.

PEARL: Besides ADHD, there are other conditions, e.g., learning problems, behavioral conditions, that can also manifest executive functioning impairment.

WHAT IS A SECTION 504 PLAN?
Case Vignette: David is a 12-year-old seventh-grade student, who was diagnosed with ADHD, combined type, in second grade. He was treated with medication and responded well. "Like night and day" his parents report, "if he takes his medication." Fortunately, he has never manifested aggressive behavior.

"Things changed when he entered middle school," parents say. "It took him a week to remember his class schedule." "And the homework problem is driving us crazy." He cannot remember what assignment is due and will not write it down, although the teacher writes it up on the blackboard. He forgets to bring home the right books, and "projects are a nightmare." "We all help him complete them on the weekend." Then he "forgets to take them to school, or if he remembers to do that he sometimes forgets to turn them in, despite the teacher's reminder as the class is being dismissed."

"Some teachers are very helpful," parents say, e.g., calling weekly or so to give them an update on what has not been turned in, whereas others refuse to cooperate at all, stating that they "can't baby David or he will never learn to be responsible." The parents wonder what their legal rights and expectations from the school are.

A. Definition
1). Section 504 is part of the Rehabilitation Act of 1973 passed by Congress to prevent discrimination against people with disabilities.
2). It is a Civil Rights Law.
3). It applies to students who have
- a physical or mental impairment (or are regarded as having such an impairment),
- an impairment that limits one or more major life activities, e.g., learning, attention.

B. Implementation
1). Implementation is primarily provision of the needed accommodations by the general education staff, but it may also include special education or related services; however, it does not, in the usual sense, provide special education services.
2). Schools do not receive federal funding for Section 504 services.

3). The aim of the Section 504 plan (accommodations) is to make certain that the student with an impairment (e.g., ADHD) has equal opportunity to be successful in the classroom as the student who does not have an impairment.

For example, students with ADHD often process information more slowly, so by giving them extra time to complete tests would mitigate against discriminating them.

C. How to obtain Section 504 accommodations
1). Parents request from school
2). Physician certifies the presence of a disability substantially limiting a major life activity (e.g., the student's ability to concentrate)
3). School documents that the disability causes an impairment

D. Examples of 504 accommodations (this is a partial list)
1). Extra time for tests
2). Extra work days for longer projects
3). Preferential seating (e.g., near the front)
4). Projects and assignments broken into shorter tasks
5). Reduced homework assignments
6). Written assignment sheets
7). Have a peer note taker to share notes
8). Teacher provides copies of lecture notes
9). A tape recorder used for lectures
10). Frequent breaks
11). Organizational assistance for time and space
12). Tests taken in a quiet room, e.g., library
13). Peer "study buddy"
14). Peer tutor
15). Extra set of books at home (to counter "forgetting")
16). Study skills class
17). Homework club after school
18). Weekly monitoring between home and school on progress, missing assignments, etc.
19). Homework tutor (at home, or an agency, where someone other than the parent [who is often "burned out"]) can be the homework overseer

PEARL: The cost of tutoring is usually paid by the parent.

E. IDEA versus Section 504 plan: Which one to choose?
1). All students qualified under IDEA can receive any of the Section 504 accommodations.
2). The reverse is not true. Section 504 is unfunded, so it provides no funds for special education.

PEARL: If a child has significant academic delays, IDEA is preferred, as it provides a wider range of programs and services, as well as IEP procedural safeguards and accountability.

CLASSROOM ACCOMMODATIONS FOR LEARNING PROBLEMS IN CHILDREN AND ADOLESCENTS WITH ADHD

A. Optimal class placement
1). Class is structured to provide clear and consistent procedures, routines, and behavior expectations
2). Both visual and auditory prompts and cues are used
3). Organizational assistance and support is provided
   • Materials
   • Workspace
   • Assignments
4). Close monitoring
5). Follow-through of the abovementioned
6). Teacher is flexible (works with student, family, and support team)
7). Teacher understands and accepts ADHD or learning disability diagnosis
8). Teacher is knowledgeable of symptoms/impairment
   • Tolerance, e.g., child not "lazy"
   • No blame
   • Empathy
9). Teacher is motivating
   • Engages child's attention and interests
   • Provides active learning
   • Provides response opportunities
   • Appreciates diversity, e.g., learning styles

PEARL: Sometimes it is very difficult to obtain the abovementioned services in a public-school classroom of 28–30 students.
   • This is why many parents will opt to send their child to a private school with fewer students, more 1:1 help.
   • If financially feasible a private school can be a great option, provided the private school offers something, e.g., smaller class size. It is better to "borrow" from the college fund to achieve success now; otherwise, college may never happen.

B. Clinician/school relationship
1). Communication is key to diagnosis and treatment, e.g., use of teacher rating scales, progress reports.

2). Identify key contact person at school (teacher, special education coordinator, nurse, counselor, etc.).

- This is particularly helpful/necessary in middle school and high school where several teachers interact with the student.
- Parents must help in facilitating this liaison.

3). Personal contact with teacher on "as-needed" basis (phone, email, etc.).

PEARL: Particularly necessary/helpful if school work is deteriorated due to noncompliance in taking medication, substance abuse, secondary diagnosis of depression, etc.

4). Clinician understands the role of the multidisciplinary team.

PEARL: If progress is not occurring, or if there is regression in school performance, a very helpful tool may be a joint meeting with the clinician, parents, and school personnel.

5). Follow-up information between school and clinician is vital (to measure medication response, functional impairment, symptoms, behavior, etc.).

PEARL: Use of rating scales (e.g., teacher Vanderbilt) or written progress reports is mandatory prior to each physician check-back appointment.

For convenience and effectiveness, it can be arranged for teachers to complete and return progress reports to the clinician online, as long as privacy is assured.

PEARL: It is necessary to get a signed release form for information to be communicated between the parents and the school. Also, depending on the student's age, and state of residence, the student's signed permission may be necessary.

PEARL: In July 2016 the US Dept. of Education classified ADHD as a "specific disability" under the Civil Rights Law (See above sections on IDEA, and Section 504).

This should greatly help our attempts to get educational accommodations for students with ADHD.

PEARL: "Supreme Court Expands Rights of Students with Disabilities" (March 2017).

The US Supreme Court ruled unanimously that children with disabilities who have school IEPs, through IDEA, must make "appropriately ambitious" educational progress.

This is due to the clause in IDEA that spells out the right of the child with a disability to a "free and appropriate education." This was a reversal of a lower court decision that stated that school districts only had to meet "minimum standards" in improvement in academic progress on the child's IEP.

Obviously, it is for the betterment of the child that the special education program strives to achieve the best outcome for the student, and not just to meet "minimum standards."

CHAPTER 3

Identifying, Screening, and Diagnosing Uncomplicated ADHD

CASE VIGNETTE: ADHD
Case 1
Robbie is a 7-year-old first grader who is brought to you by the parents because the school said they "couldn't keep him in class unless he got help." He was kicked off the bus the first week for not staying in his seat. In the class room, he gets up and walks around, talks out loud, and disrupts the class. He refuses to do any work and says he "won't" when the teacher asks him to sit down.

On the playground, he has had some fight with peers, who refuse to let him play in their games because he changes the rules.

Robbie started kindergarten shortly after turning 5 years. After 2 weeks, he was removed from school, as he was "not ready." Subsequently, he completed kindergarten but with great difficulty due to overactivity and behavior outbursts.

His dad reports that he had similar issues as a child but "outgrew them."

Case 2
Mary is a 12-year-old seventh grader who has done well in school, say her parents, until this current year (7th grade). She is described as "sweet, smart, and fun to be around." She has always said that school has been "easy" for her, and she enjoys school greatly, mostly because of her friends.

This year she entered middle school and now says she "doesn't like school." She refuses to do her homework. In addition, she has complained a lot about headaches, which have caused her to miss several days of classes. She has an appointment scheduled with a neurologist to look into that.

Her vocational goal is to become a pediatrician, but her parents are pessimistic about that, given the recent change of events.

AAP Clinical Practice Guidelines for the Diagnosis, Evaluation, and Treatment of ADHD in Children and Adolescents: 2011 (summarized and paraphrased).

Diagnosis

1. Any child between the ages 4 and 18 years who presents to the clinician with academic or behavioral issues, such as inattention, hyperactivity, or impulsivity, should be assessed for ADHD.
2. The clinician should use established criteria, including signs or symptoms causing impairment, in at least two settings, e.g., home and school, after obtaining information from parents, teachers, or other caregivers.
3. Other conditions should also be assessed, e.g., anxiety, depression, learning disabilities (if indicated), behavior disorders (such as oppositional defiant disorder or conduct disorder), and hearing, vision, or other health problems, all of which can mimic ADHD or be coexistent with an ADHD diagnosis.
4. The clinician should be aware that ADHD is a chronic medical condition and therefore the child/adolescent with ADHD should be treated as any other child who has special healthcare needs, utilizing the chronic care model.

DEFINITION OF ADHD
ADHD is a neurodevelopmental disorder with three cardinal traits: inattention, hyperactivity, and impulsivity.
1) The inattentive traits include behaviors such as problems sustaining attention, losing things, weak organizational skills, and poor time management.
2) The hyperactive and impulsive traits include behaviors such as being fidgety or wiggly (or outright hyperactive), impatient, noisy, and blurting out inappropriately.
3) The traits must be persistent over time, e.g., 6 months at least; must have occurred in two or more settings; must be impairing to the child; and must not be due to another medical condition.

PEARL: The Vanderbilt rating scales (see Chapter 1), although not diagnostic in and of themselves, are a great initial screening tool for assessing children and adolescents on the possibility of an ADHD diagnosis (also, they are free online).

ADHD is the most common neurodevelopmental disorder that a primary care physician will encounter in the office setting. Its estimated incidence is about 10% in children (about 200 kids in an average panel of 2000 patients).

Question: How many kids are identified, diagnosed, and undergoing treatment in your practice?

Developmental course of ADHD (possible symptoms at progressive ages, not all symptoms seen in every child) is presented in the following.

- Pregnancy: Increased total activity in utero.
- Birth to 1 year: Prolonged irritability, may last for 9—12 months, rather than usual 3 months colic.
- 2—4 Years: Usually persistent 2-year-old behavior, e.g., overactive, impulsive.
- 4—6 Years: May be expelled from preschool because of overactivity, "can't sit still during circle time," and may hit, bite, push, kick, etc.
- 6—12 Years (elementary school): Hyperactive; out of seat; loud, boisterous, blurts out; bothers peers; unable to get work done; needs 1:1 monitoring; fights on playground; rarely invited to parties; few, if any, friends; sleep disorder (falling asleep, "night owl," hard to awaken); needs 1:1 to get ready for school, may be tardy; misses school bus.
- Increased incidence of enuresis/encopresis, falls behind at school (below grade level), fine motor problems in two-thirds of patients, gross motor problems in one-third of patients, "daredevil" behavior, poor self-esteem.
- 12—18 Years (adolescence): Continuation of many of the abovementioned issues.

School failure often due to not doing homework or projects, claims "too boring."

Lack of friends; immature socially.

Oppositional (excessive from normal).

May need to do summer school.

Needs 1:1 help to complete homework.

Poor coordination, resists practice and team rules so dislikes team sports; does better with individual sports, e.g., martial arts.

Risk behaviors: drugs (e.g., pot), ethyl alcohol (ETOH), sex, delinquency, reckless driving.

May develop other coexistent problems, e.g., anxiety, depression, conduct disorder.

- Adult: Less than expected educational achievement, e.g., does not graduate high school or attend college; marital difficulties; domestic violence; diverse chronic substance abuse (ETOH, tobacco, etc.)

Job dysfunction: Frequent changes, impulse control, conflict with peers, bosses, etc.

Troubles with the law, e.g., traffic violations, accidents, driving under the influence.

DIAGNOSIS

Early diagnosis and treatment is associated with better outcomes (preschool diagnosis and treatment will be discussed in chapter 5).

Rule: Any child with significant behavioral or academic concerns in the early years of schooling should be screened for ADHD.

The reason? There is a significant likelihood that ADHD is the cause. However, simply obtaining an ADHD rating scale is inadequate to make the diagnosis of ADHD.

Rule: Positive ADHD rating scales are not a definitive diagnosis of ADHD.

ADHD rating scales merely denote, in a quantitative measure, the presence or absence of ADHD traits. There are many other diagnoses that could result in a rating scale suggestive of ADHD. These include conditions in four different categories: medical, developmental, family/environmental, and mental. These are called ADHD "look-alikes" because they may also produce symptoms suggesting ADHD and must, therefore, be ruled out.

Rule: If a child has a (+) ADHD rating scale, other possible etiologies must be ruled out (a thorough history and physical examination [PE] will rule out most of them).

Examples of conditions that may have ADHD-like symptoms.

Medical
  Genetic (familial ADHD): the condition we refer to as "ADHD"
  Prematurity
  Neonatal CNS, hypoxia, etc.
  Small for gestational age (intra-uterine growth retardation)
  Near drowning
  Traumatic brain injury/CNS infections
  Sleep apnea or other sleep disorders, such as premature awakening, restless legs, nocturnal enuresis, excessive movement
  Lead intoxication
  Syndromes (fetal alcohol syndrome, Turner syndrome, fragile X syndrome, Williams syndrome, etc.)
  Chronic illness
  Medication side effects, e.g., allergy or seizure medication
  Vision/hearing disorders
  History of iron deficiency with/without anemia
Developmental
  Low/borderline IQ
  Learning disabilities/dyslexia
  Autistic spectrum disorders
  Speech/language disorders

Mental health conditions
    Anxiety and/or depression
    Bipolar disorder
    Reactive attachment disorder
    Oppositional defiant disorder
    Conduct disorder
    Obsessive compulsive disorder
    Disruptive mood dysregulation disorder
Family/environmental
    Family dysfunction (separation, death, divorce, inadequate parenting, etc.)
    Sexual abuse
    Physical/mental abuse or neglect
    Environments producing aggression

Obviously, it takes more than a rating scale to sort all this out. To start, it is necessary to take a thorough medical history including the following (if this is a child from your own medical practice, most of this information will be already known to you or available in the medical record):

1) Medical history
   - Pregnancy, delivery, chronic use of medication during pregnancy (acetaminophen, seizure medication)
   - Infancy (colic, etc.)
   - Serious illnesses, injuries, hospitalizations
   - Review of systems
   - Developmental landmarks
2) Genetic/family history
   - Learning problems
   - Dyslexia
   - ADHD
   - Bipolar disorder
   - Autism
   - Anxiety/depression
   - Other syndromes
3) Developmental/educational history
   - Preschool history, questionable problems
   - School history (behavior, academic)
   - Grades—report cards
   - Speech/language issues, treatment
   - School or private academic testing
   - Homework completion
   - Tutoring
4) Social history
   - Friends
   - Invitations to parties, etc.
   - Sports activities (team vs. individual)
   - Likes/dislikes, hobbies
5) Family history
   - One versus two parents
   - Sibling relationships

- Foster child/adopted?
- Separation/divorce
- Custody
- Living arrangements
- After-school environment

Almost all this information can be obtained using a parent questionnaire so that the parent appointment can concentrate on the ADHD concerns, behaviors, etc. by using, e.g., the Academic and/or Behavioral Concerns Parent Questionnaire provided in Chapter 1.

Important: Ask the parents to mention two or three of their child's best skills or traits (this will be important when designing a treatment program).

The next thing is to do a complete PE and a brief neurologic examination, particularly stressing the following:

PE
- Height, weight (percentiles, body mass index)
- Pulse, blood pressure
- Vision and hearing screening
- Signs/symptoms of chronic illness
- Dysmorphic features
- Others, e.g., tics or other physical abnormalities that may affect school and/or behavior

Neurologic examination (for skills that will impact school [e.g., writing], social activities, sports, etc.)
- Mental status: Is he/she developmentally appropriate?
- Brief neurologic screening
- Hand/foot/eye dominance
- Gross motor (gait, balance, skip, hop, throw a ball, etc.)
- Fine motor (tie shoes, write name, draw a picture, etc.)

Following the PE/neurologic examinations the child should be interviewed alone.

1) Child/adolescent interview
   - Perception of why he/she is here
   - Inquire about

School:	Like/dislike, easy/hard, boring/fun; subjects liked/disliked
Social:	Friends, sleepovers, parties
Family:	Describe parents, siblings, rules, chores
Likes/dislikes:	Hobbies, sports
Vocation	

- Possible use of "three wishes" technique (ages 6–12 years). Tell the child that you are a pretend fairy godmother and will grant three wishes. What would they be?
- Possible "draw a person" technique of himself or herself or family (ages 6–12 years)

2) Observe
- Activity level, signs or symptoms of ADHD (**PEARL:** Sometimes children who are very hyperactive in the classroom will not be the same in the examination room. Do not be fooled into saying "he/she doesn't have ADHD.")
- Evidence of mood disorder, anxiety, depression
- Evidence of communication problems: Autistic spectrum, unusual comments or behavior, eye contact, difficulty with articulation, stuttering, etc.
- Evidence of dysmorphology
- Estimation of IQ

PEARL: Remember, your estimate may be inaccurate in children with language impairment, or who are socially "bright."
- Write name (fine motor)

Diagnostic Tests to Consider

1) Hemoglobin/hematocrit test: If not done recently, it is done to rule out (R/O) anemia as a potential cause of inattention, usually in a teenager, e.g., due to menses in a girl, but poor eating habits as well (boys).
2) Electroencephalography: If there is a history of "spacing out," it is done to R/O petit mal epilepsy, or if the history suggests psychomotor seizures.
3) Chromosome karyotyping and DNA analysis for fragile X syndrome if examination suggests dysmorphology.
4) Blood lead test: Use "high-risk" approach (environmental exposure, old home/lead paint).
5) Substance abuse test
6) Psychoeducational test: If significant academic delays, e.g., >6 months below grade level, occur, it is done to R/O learning disability as either the primary diagnosis or secondary diagnosis with ADHD; it requires 1:1 testing by a school or private psychologist (this is discussed in more detail in Chapter 2). Many children being assessed for ADHD will not have a significant academic delay (>6 months) and therefore will not need a complete psychoeducational evaluation.
7) Occupational and/or physical therapy consultation (for fine and gross motor skills impairment).
8) Brain scan: Examples are CT, MRI, positron emission tomography, and single-photon emission computed tomography. Currently, scans are useful only for research purposes and are NOT INDICATED in the usual diagnostic evaluation for ADHD (exception: history of seizures or other chronic neurologic issues, e.g., traumatic brain injury, etc.).
9) Computerized diagnostic tools are TOO INACCURATE to be used solely for diagnosis of ADHD.

How to obtain information, and what type of information to obtain, from schools.

1) Teacher(s) complete Vanderbilt rating scales.
2) Parents should bring in all the report cards since kindergarten for review, with particular attention to the teacher comments, not just the grades.
3) Review results of any testing/evaluations done by school personnel (parent and older child need to sign the release form). Also review from any private psychoeducational evaluations.
4) **PEARL:** Talk personally to the teacher. This can be invaluable (and, given the current availability of voicemail, can almost always be arranged. The information from an experienced teacher can be an invaluable resource to the diagnostic process).
5) In some instances, having a school counselor or psychologist do a classroom observation and report back to you can also be a very helpful resource, e.g., regarding behavior, focus, and work completion.

How should all this information be obtained, organized, and pulled together? Several options can be utilized depending on the practice setting and style.

Examples:

1) Parents call in to the clinician's office and his or her concern is screened by the office nurse or the ADHD coordinator, who then, if appropriate, sets up the ADHD diagnostic process.

or

2) Parents come in for a brief 10- to 15-min appointment with the clinician, who then, if appropriate, triggers the diagnostic process.
3) If appropriate, parents then receive a packet containing teacher and parent ADHD rating scales, Academic and/or Behavioral Concerns Parent Questionnaire, and release forms to be signed for reports from other agencies, sources, etc.

Parents should bring in for review all the report cards (if available) from kindergarten through 12th grade and other progress reports, outside evaluations, etc.

Optimally, all the abovementioned will then be available for review prior to the first appointment.

4) Parent intake can be from 30 to 60 min (one or two appointments), depending on the complexity of the problem, how well the child is known to the practice, and how much material needs to be reviewed and discussed.
5) The child PE/neurologic examination and 1:1 interview in our clinic takes 30–60 min (one or two

appointments) and is more appropriately done at a separate appointment from parent intake (often for reimbursement issues). Each clinic obviously can develop their own system and approach to the intake appointment process.

Note: In our specialized center for ADHD, we were able to schedule 60-min appointments, as we were a referral center. In a general medical clinic that may not be possible, so 30-min appointments will be necessary. Overall, an ADHD assessment from start to finish in our center usually entailed about 3–4 h of clinic appointment time. This could be shortened, perhaps even to 2 h or so, in the private office setting, when patients are known to the clinic and a medical chart is already available.

6) Final summary appointment or appointments: This involves review of all information received, a diagnostic formulation, and development of a treatment plan.
   • Sometimes the summary appointment becomes more of a "progress" appointment, pending more information (e.g., psychoeducational evaluation, consultations from neurology, genetics, and psychiatry) before a more specific diagnosis and treatment plan is formulated.
   • Adolescents would be expected to be involved in this discussion, although in some situations parents may wish to speak privately as well.
   • With younger children, their involvement in the discussion should be discussed between parents and the clinician.

Certainly, if treatment for ADHD is being recommended, particularly medication, the child definitively needs to be told (at his/her level) about the diagnosis and purpose of therapy, especially to avoid misconceptions regarding any medicine.

Common Errors in Diagnosis

1) Inadequate history—too brief, use of one source (e.g., parent) rather than two sources of information (e.g., include school).
2) Overreliance on rating scales.
3) Using "broadband" rating scales (e.g., Child Behavior Checklist or Behavior Assessment System for Children) that screen for ADHD issues only superficially.
4) Using the response to medication as a diagnostic test (not all ADHD is responsive to any given medication). Likewise the absence of response does not R/O ADHD.
5) Not assessing for coexisting conditions, e.g., anxiety, depression, and learning disabilities, which are not only ADHD "look-alikes" but also often coexist with

ADHD, and treatment of the ADHD and not treating the coexistent condition will not produce a successful outcome.

ASSESSING FOR ADHD IN THE HOMESCHOOLED CHILD

1) This can be a real challenge, for example, obtaining information from at least two sources.
2) Here are some suggestions:
   • Perhaps there is some prior school information to access. For example, the child was removed from the classroom because he/she was overactive, disruptive, and parents refused the advice to have an assessment. Review any previous report cards.
3) Have a visiting nurse (health department) make a home visit to evaluate parenting style, behavior in home, etc.
4) Enroll the child in a group setting (e.g., social skills class) to get more information regarding behavior, attentiveness, etc.
5) Get information from another adult in the child's life, such as a soccer coach, a Boy Scout leader.
6) Do a learning assessment (through school, if possible) that may document inattention, overactivity, distractibility, and impulsivity and may help in ruling out a learning disorder.
7) Resist using a "trial of medication" as a diagnostic test. Positive response or lack of a response does not prove or rule out anything.

PEARL: In light of the news regarding the Flint, Michigan, water supply, we all need to remember that lead can be a rare cause of not only ADHD but also learning and behavior problems and decrease in IQ. Studies have shown increased levels of lead in other regions of the United States as well, which tend to be in poverty areas, where there is still old lead paint on homes. DO YOU KNOW ANY SUCH AREAS IN YOUR COMMUNITY?

The only truly "safe" level of lead in the blood is zero.

>5 μg, Concern
>10 μg, Serious

OTHER COMMON COEXISTING CONDITIONS SEEN IN CHILDREN AND ADOLESCENTS WITH ADHD

We have already discussed the major coexistent conditions commonly seen in children/adolescents with ADHD, namely,
• oppositional defiant disorder, ~50% (males);
• learning disabilities, ~30%;

- conduct disorder, ~20%;
- anxiety, ~25%;
- depression, 5%–50% (depending on the type, major depression vs. dysthymia);
- bipolar disorder.

Examples of other common, although usually less impairing, coexisting conditions are discussed in the following.

- Sleep disorders: 90%, mostly insomnia.
- Gross motor coordination problems: ~ 30%. For this reason many children with ADHD are not very good athletes, and along with all the rules and practices and "downtime" associated with being on a team, they do not like team sports (however, there are always exceptions, e.g., Michael Phelps). They should be encouraged in individual sports, such as martial arts, bike riding, swimming. Overzealous fathers should be prevented from pushing their children with ADHD into team sports if they are reluctant.
- Fine motor coordination problems: ~ 65%. Physicians once used these subtle fine motor signs, called "soft neurologic signs," to help them aid in the diagnosis of ADHD; however, we now realize that they are not specific to ADHD, but occur in many other conditions, even in normal children. However, it is important to recognize them because they sometimes have neurologic effects on the child, which might have to be taken into account in the treatment program, e.g., effect on fine motor/writing skills.
- Enuresis.
- Encopresis (stool withholding).

PEARL: When you see encopresis, look for ADHD.

In addition, writing is very difficult for most children with ADHD. Writing is a very difficult task to achieve because it requires several skills such as short-term memory recall, fine motor coordination, space management, and remembering all the "rules" regarding what constitutes a sentence, paragraph, capitalization, punctuation.

PEARL: Writing can be very stressful, and it requires a lot of practice like having the child write a "journal" daily, even if only one sentence. (e.g., what was the best thing that happened to you today?). Interestingly, teachers sometimes report that the handwriting of a child with ADHD becomes more legible when the child takes ADHD medication. I suspect the reason for this is that the illegibility is due to hurried, careless, sloppy handwriting and the medication improves the underlying impulsivity so that the child writes less hurriedly and more clearly. On the other hand, if medication does not improve the legibility, it is probably a fine motor issue, which could be helped by a referral to occupational therapy.

Also written reports to the teacher should be replaced occasionally by oral reports (e.g., book reports) (to give the child a "break").

PEARL: Here's a zebra! NICHD (National Institute of Child Health and Human Development) Maya Lodish, MD.

Pheochromocytomas and paragangliomas (both rare tumors) can masquerade and present with ADHD symptoms.

The possible clue? An increased blood pressure.

Another reason why we should always take kids' blood pressures.

CHAPTER 4

General Principles of Multimodality Treatments for Children and Adolescents With Uncomplicated ADHD

AMERICAN ACADEMY OF PEDIATRICS GUIDELINES FOR ADHD TREATMENT

1. Treatment varies according to patient
   a) In preschool children (4–5 years), initial treatment should be parent and/or teacher applied behavior therapy.

      If the behavior therapy does not successfully control the symptoms a medication trial using small doses of methylphenidate (e.g., 2.5 mg bid) may be initiated after weighing the risk of possible benefits with potential side effects (weight loss, sleep disturbance, etc.), along with the negative effects on the child's development, if left untreated.
   b) In elementary-school children the clinician should prescribe FDA-approved ADHD medication and/or approved behavior therapy (by both teacher and parent), along with appropriate accommodations in the classroom.
   c) For adolescents, FDA-approved medication should be initiated and other behavioral and/or academic accommodations should be made as necessary.
2. Medication dose should be titrated upward to achieve maximal benefit with minimal side effects. Note: These guidelines will be revised in 2017/2018. ADHD treatment requires a multimodality approach that includes
   1) parent and child/youth education about ADHD,
   2) academic accommodations,
   3) behavior therapy,
   4) usually, specific medication.

   The goals of ADHD treatment are
   1) to alleviate the core symptoms of ADHD;
   2) to lessen accompanying behaviors, e.g., oppositional defiant disorder (ODD);
   3) to achieve improved peer relationships;
   4) to enhance academic success;
   5) to recognize and treat coexistent conditions;
   6) to reduce high-risk behavior, e.g., substance abuse;
   7) to improve organizational skills (i.e., executive function);
   8) to enhance self-esteem;
   9) to assure progression into functional adulthood;
   10) to improve family interactions.

   From these goals, it is apparent that using only one specific therapy, e.g., medications, will not assure every goal is met.

   For example, medication is the best treatment for reducing the core symptoms of ADHD, but it only partly helps in treating ODD and does not improve executive functioning impairment to any significant degree.

   Let us look next at the specific types of treatment for ADHD. Only two treatments have significant evidence base to support them: behavior therapy and specific medications. The other two components of ADHD multimodal treatment are parent and patient education about ADHD and school or job interventions. So let us discuss what is involved.
   1) Patient and parent (caregiver) education regarding what is known currently about ADHD, i.e., cause or causes, how it was diagnosed and treated, prognosis, and benefits and risks of treatment.
      This education is begun with parents and child/youth at the summary appointment, but often there is not enough time to cover all that is needed to know.
      Fortunately, there are many resources:
      • Books—A whole resource list is included later in the chapter for books specifically designed for small children, teenagers, caregivers and parents, and teachers.

- Internet—Much is available but, like all subjects, a great deal is nonscientific. Child and parents need to be directed to those websites that promote accurate and evidence-based information (see the list on Resources).
- Local and national organizations—For example, the Children and Adults with Attention-Deficit/ Hyperactivity Disorder (CHADD) web page **www.chadd.org** is an outstanding resource supporting not only evidence-based treatment but also wonderful information regarding behavior therapy and medication, research, prognosis, monitoring, and advocacy.
- Other organizations listed in parent resources—CHADD has a national meeting for parents, educators, and clinicians. There are many local chapters as well for parents to hear guest speakers discuss various aspects of ADHD treatment. Also, the Learning Disabilities Association of America has similar offerings, as well as tutoring resources and a web page. Sylvan Centers can also be a tutoring resource.

2) The second component of multimodal care for ADHD involves academic accommodations. In Chapter 5, subsection ADHD Goes to College, there is a list of ways ADHD presents challenges in school in addition to its core symptoms, which are inattention, hyperactivity, and impulsivity. These challenges fall into three types:
   a) executive function, e.g., organization, time management, study skills, completing assignments;
   b) social/behavioral skills including peer relationships, handling stress, anger, and frustration;
   c) following instructions and rules.

No wonder children with ADHD fall behind in school. We know that about 12% or so of developing children typically qualify for an educational diagnosis of specific learning disorder (~2 standard deviation below the mean for age and IQ). Many kids with ADHD do not qualify for special education under those strict criteria in the Individuals with Disabilities Education Act (IDEA) that provides for special education. So how can they be helped? Fortunately, there is another category in IDEA for children who have a medical condition (such as asthma, heart defect, ADHD) that impairs school performance because of symptoms, absenteeism, etc. This category is called "Other Health Impaired." Under this category the child with ADHD may receive special education help. Unfortunately, schools have some leeway in determining who gets help under this category.

So it is not always a "slam dunk." But if the child with ADHD has academic delays, it is always worth a try.

PEARL: The recent decision by the U.S. Dept. of Education to classify ADHD as a "specific disability" should also make it more likely to have special education services available to children with ADHD.

However, we have another "ace up our sleeve." It is called Section 504 of the Civil Rights Act. This law prevents discrimination against persons with a disability, and, fortunately, the federal government also classifies ADHD as an "educational handicap," which it really is. As this is a Civil Rights law, it has no money attached for special education, as does IDEA. What it does do is guarantee certain accommodations by the school for the child under the ruling that if those accommodations were not provided, there would be discrimination to the child with ADHD. These accommodations might include
1) preferential seating (toward the front);
2) extra time for tests or projects;
3) written assignment sheets in advance, e.g., weekly;
4) second set of books to keep at home;
5) attending a study skills class (where a teacher is available for brief help such as clarification of homework instruction);
6) homework "club" after school for an hour or so where a teacher is available for assistance with homework completion;
7) tests given in a quiet room (e.g., library);
8) weekly communication with the parent (voicemail, progress report, etc.);
9) "grace period" provided, e.g., 24-h "grace" for handing in homework without penalty or 3- to 4-day "grace" for longer assignments or projects, in case they are finished but "forgot to bring them."

These are only a few of the Section 504 accommodations but are the most helpful and commonly used (the parent books, e.g., by Sandra Rief and Chris Dendy, listed in the Resources chapter 18 are loaded with suggestions).

Rule: Almost every, if not every, adolescent with ADHD, in my experience, should have a 504 plan, unless he/she is already covered under IDEA.

How does one qualify for a 504 plan?

Parents request it.

Childs medical doctor has to verify the diagnosis (ADHD).

The school has to verify that ADHD is causing an impairment to the child's academic progress.

A Section 504 plan is a very powerful instrument for the parent and child in that failure of the school to provide what was promised in the 504 plan is "violation of the child's civil rights."

The final two components of multimodal care for ADHD are the only treatments that are evidence based.

3) Behavior therapy

First, let us mention what types of therapy are either not helpful at all or minimally helpful.

a) Play therapy, e.g., the counselor/therapist may play checkers or a board game with the child with ADHD. There is no significant evidence this has ever been helpful for ADHD treatment.

PEARL: Make sure your patient is not receiving play therapy (probably waste of time and money).

b) Anger classes, e.g., by a well-intentioned school counselor who gathers several kids with ADHD for a weekly group meeting. This is probably minimally helpful. Kids with ADHD almost always know cognitively that anger outbursts can be misdirected or wrong. What they need to do is to learn and practice within their social environment how to appropriately express their anger/frustration in a nonaggressive or nondestructive manner. This is done best in a small-group setting, with close monitoring by adult(s), where inappropriate behavior is immediately recognized and an intervention made (sort of an on-the-job training).

PEARL: Before discussing the specific forms of behavior therapy, let us discuss some general concepts of what we want to achieve with our behavior program and how to achieve those goals.

c) Appropriate behavior: There should be well-established house rules and expectations in place. Chaos breeds more chaos.

d) Good behavior maximized: Good behavior should always be acknowledged with praise.

e) Bad behavior minimized: Annoying behavior should usually be ignored, if mild, so as to not call attention to it, unless it is harmful, dangerous, or destructive (which then not only should be acknowledged but also may result in a consequence).

f) Compliance with requests: Commands and/or directives should always be developmentally age appropriate.

g) Good behavior in public: Always have a plan-ahead discussion regarding expectations prior to visiting a public place.

h) Effective discipline: Discipline must be consistent, appropriate to the misbehavior, and effective.

4) Examples of appropriate forms of behavior therapy in ADHD treatment. Most are familiar to average families but need to be intensified in children with ADHD.

• Time out.

PEARL: Have parents read the book "SOS Help for Parents" (see the list under the title Resources).

• Token economies: In this system a poker chip or marble of one color is used to reward good behavior and an opposite color is used for inappropriate behavior.

A predetermined number of accumulated chips/marbles result in a modest reward, e.g., more TV or game time.

Negative marbles/chips can be worked off by doing extra chores, etc.

Variation: Reward chips cannot be turned in or redeemed until all or some of the negative ones are paid off.

Very effective system. Very visual, matter of fact, and black and white to modify or prevent arguing with the child; works for many/most children with ADHD.

• 1-2-3 Magic: A behavior system designed by Dr. Tom Phelan (handbook and video, sometimes can be rented at the library). Some clinics buy several copies of the video and/or book and "loan" them to families.

This is based on the concept of "three strikes—you're out," with progressive warnings and finally an intervention. VERY EFFECTIVE FOR MOST CHILDREN WITH ADHD AND AGED <12 YEARS.

• Small-group environments, with high adult-to-child ratio, e.g., one adult to three or so children, where inappropriate behavior is immediately recognized and an intervention made.

Examples: Special behavior classroom or special summer camp program for kids with ADHD (most summer recreational programs for sports or other activities do not offer much help because the child-to-adult ratio is too high).

PEARL: The abovementioned scenarios can also be very helpful behavior therapy in a positive way by the use of a technique called "catching them when they're good," in which the child is "caught" by the adult doing something positive behaviorally and is immediately complimented and rewarded.

• School Daily Report Card

One at a time, inappropriate behaviors, such as blurting out, are identified. Through observation the number of usual infractions is identified, e.g., 10 times per day (blurting out).

Weekly goals are established, e.g., first-week goal is no more than seven episodes per day. Each day the goal is reached, it equals a star. Obtaining the prescribed number of stars (predetermined) results in a modest reward (more video time, not a new bike!).

In the subsequent weeks the goal is lowered, e.g., from seven to four episodes. After a few weeks the inappropriate behavior becomes infrequent or is extinguished totally. Then move on to the next goal (negative behavior).

Teacher keeps track of the progress and violations and sends a note home to the parent, who gives out rewards when earned.

It is a very helpful system and can be used both at school and at home.

PEARL: It works on only one inappropriate behavior at a time.

Option: Some parents need/want a behavior expert/counselor (e.g., child psychologist) to help with or choose from the above types of therapy. This can be a very helpful, although somewhat expensive, option. Many books and websites in the Resources Chapter can walk the parents through these techniques step by step.

MEDICATION THERAPY

This section will deal with the general concepts of medication management, treatment of common side effects, etc. We will mention, although not recommend, specific brand names, but not discuss medicines that are not FDA approved (a subsequent section in this current chapter, ADHD Alternative/Complementary Treatments, discusses therapies including herbs, vitamins, other supplements, or techniques that have no significant scientific data to support their usage and that, in some cases, are potentially harmful to the child).

Medication treatment was first "discovered" by Dr. Bradley in 1937, a psychiatrist who was working in an institution. He gave Benzedrine (a type of stimulant medicine similar to amphetamine) to several children in an institutional setting who suffered from postencephalitic symptoms of aggressiveness and hyperactivity. The reason for giving Benzedrine was to treat allergy symptoms. There was dramatic improvement in the hyperactivity and aggressiveness in many of the children who received Benzedrine. This response was immediately noted in the field of child psychiatry.

Quote by Dr. Bradley (*American Journal of Psychiatry,* 1937):

"To see a single dose of Benzedrine produce a greater improvement in school performance than the combined effects of a capable staff working in a most favorable setting, would have been all but demoralizing to the teachers, had not the improvement been so gratifying from a practical viewpoint."

After World War II, in the late 1940s and early 1950s, research was done that demonstrated the validity of Dr. Bradley's observation that "stimulant" medication, e.g., the amphetamines and later methylphenidate, had a pronounced effect on some children who struggled in school with sitting still, paying attention, and completing their work, what we now refer to as the "core symptoms of ADHD, i.e., hyperactivity, inattention, and impulsivity."

So since that time, stimulant medications consisting of amphetamines and methylphenidate in a variety of dosage types and brand names have been the mainstay of ADHD treatment.

Medications are often the single most helpful treatment you can offer to a child with ADHD. Should they be used alone for treatment? Absolutely not! As mentioned earlier, the goals of ADHD treatment in kids are very diverse, and medications, although the best treatment for the "core symptoms," are only minimally helpful for treating other symptoms, or not at all for others.

PEARL: So medications are important along with the other aspects of multimodal treatment, which includes behavior therapy, parent/child education, and school accommodations.

PEARL: The Multimodal Treatment Study of Children with ADHD (MTA) and other studies have shown that the best treatment of ADHD in kids is a combined therapy of medications and behavior therapy (see later chapter 18, section Hallmark Studies regarding the MTA study referenced above. Read it!). Unfortunately, numerous studies have documented that most children/adolescents with ADHD are receiving only medication therapy.

What are the problems with medication treatment?
1) Side effects: Stimulant medications have many side effects that must be dealt with proactively or promptly. Fortunately, serious or life-threatening side effects are very rare as to be essentially nonexistent.
2) Overreliance on medication due to its high effectiveness and the exclusion of the other components of multimodal therapy.
3) Medication abuse or diversion: In our experience, kids with ADHD are less likely to abuse their medication for self-use, but they may alter the

dosage without talking to their doctor. What they are more likely to do is divert or sell their medications to others. Hence, the most widely abused medication in the United States is Adderall (long-acting amphetamine), both to "get high" and to "cram for exams." Safeguards must be in place to prevent this.

4) Lack of compliance (why?)
   - Side effects not dealt with
   - Wrong dosage
   - Improper monitoring
   - Lack of effect
   - Inadequate trial
   - Peer pressure

Preparation for a Trial of Medications

Make a list of several symptoms that occur commonly in ADHD but may be caused or worsened by medications (make a list for each child prior to initiation of ADHD medication to check whether a symptom was new onset since medication started or represents worsening of prior symptoms, e.g., insomnia).

Examples: Headache, stomach ache, insomnia, loss of appetite, irritability, tiredness, tics, seizures, behavioral rebound (late afternoon after school is let out), and aggressiveness.

PEARL: For the patient who is to start medications write down all these symptoms occurring at baseline on a list or chart, denoting the frequency, severity, time of day, etc. This will provide a baseline for comparing symptoms after initiation of medication.

Rule: Measure and record height, weight, pulse, and blood pressure (BP) before onset of medication trial and during all subsequent visits.

Medication Trials: Initiate, Review, Refine

1) If possible always start with stimulants: Any stimulant you try will be 70% effective, and if one type is not successful or tolerated switch to the other type. There is a 90% success rate for stimulants if both types are utilized (amphetamine vs. methylphenidate).

Which stimulant to choose? Consider the following factors:
   - Duration of action: 4, 8, or 12 h, e.g., teens need evening coverage for homework completion
   - Availability: for example, what does the patient's insurance plan cover?
   - Family history: for example, has a sibling responded to a certain medication?
   - Side-effect profile: for example, methylphenidates maybe less likely to affect appetite than amphetamines. Same with sleep.
   - If possible, try to use single AM dose.

PEARL: Your familiarity with the medication. Best to regularly use three or four medications, rather than six to eight different medications, to gain more experience and comfort in their usage.
   - Ability to swallow pills: Can the pill be opened and dissolved in liquid, e.g., Vyvanse versus Concerta? Or use a liquid or chewable form, which is available now.

PEARL: Usually it is OK to start with the generic form, if available, but if there is no response then brand name may be tried before giving up on a specific medication. Like all medications, generic medications usually work OK, but FDA has recently removed two generic stimulant medications from the market because of lack of documented effectiveness.

2) In general, start with either 8- or 12-h medication (exception is preschoolers, which will be discussed later).

3) Start with the lowest dose possible and titrate upward at 5- to 7-day intervals, but preferably no longer in most cases (need to reach optimal dose in 4 weeks or less).

4) Monitor weekly, e.g., a phone call to the clinic using the teacher and parent rating scales such as Vanderbilt, along with the feedback regarding behavioral changes and side effects (written follow-up via rating scales is superior to verbal ones such as "doing better").

PEARL: Preschool children with ADHD (see chapter ADHD Pre-school) need to be seen weekly initially.

5) Continue to titrate upward until no further improvement is noticed, intolerable side effects occur, or maximum dosage is reached. Examples of maximum dosages: (in general, not a hard-and-fast rule)
   amphetamines, 1 mg/kg per day
   methylphenidate, 2 mg/kg per day

PEARL: Remember that Focalin, a methylphenidate, is twice as strong as other methylphenidates, as it is a pure dextro isomer, and all other methylphenidates are a mixture of dextro and levo isomers (dextro isomer is the active ingredient).

6) Most children need 12 h of medication coverage, provided by a single AM dose if possible. Worsening insomnia would require an 8-h medication.

7) Medication by and large should be used 365 d/year, especially on weekends because ADHD does not remit on holidays and weekends (see the section How to Manage Side Effects of Stimulants).

8) If there has been a weekly phone follow-up for the first 2–3 weeks, as well as use of parent and teacher rating scales to measure improvement in symptoms, a check-back appointment should

occur NO LATER THAN 1 MONTH after initiation of medication (If poor phone and teacher follow-up then see the child back earlier.)

9) Presumably then, if things are going satisfactorily, check-back appointments should be scheduled at 3-month intervals. Research has documented that at least four visits per year are needed for optimal management (see MTA) to anticipate complications such as growth spurt and the need for dosage increase before symptoms get out of control. Also, growth should be monitored at 3-month intervals.

   Sometimes adolescents whose symptoms are well controlled, who are good at self-monitoring and compliance, and whose dosage has been stable with no significant coexisting conditions can be followed at 6-month intervals, but these are usually an exception to the rule. Remember, things can deteriorate quickly in an adolescent (discussed later), requiring immediate assessment.

10) In adolescents, monitoring ADHD can often be more reliable by using school report cards and progress reports rather than using teacher rating scales, which are less accurate in adolescent patients because of the volume of students with whom the teacher interacts.

11) Most adolescents with ADHD can be treated with a single medication unless coexistent conditions (e.g., Anxiety or Depression) require additional medications (e.g., a selective serotonin reuptake inhibitor).

12) It is unlikely that any adolescent who takes ADHD medications will be able to control symptoms adequately off medications prior to completion of high school, and most likely not until 1–2 years of college. A proactive discussion on this should be started early in the treatment course.

13) Children and adolescents should be reminded that once school has ended and a vocational career is reached, about 90% of patients find medication no longer necessary. This is mostly due to interest and motivation in the new career, the burden of school being removed, and the child learning coping skills. Also, we know that in many patients the ADHD symptoms actually do remit slowly over time, so that in adult life they are much less prominent, perhaps even sub-threshold (however, the fallouts including coexistent problems such as anxiety, depression, and marital and job dysfunction might now be the dominant concerns).

14) Neither stimulant medications nor the α-agonists and atomoxetine need periodic laboratory data of any type.

How to Manage Side Effects of Stimulants
See also the Case Scenarios section.
1) Headache/stomach ache: Not unusual for the first 2 weeks and usually mild. Try to "ride it out." If too severe and persistent, then discontinue medication and try something else (e.g., a different stimulant).
2) Decreased appetite/poor or inadequate weight gain: COMMON SIDE EFFECTS!
   - Dose during or after meals, e.g., breakfast.
   - Take high-calorie snacks in the afternoon and during bedtime.
   - Encourage "grazing." Bedtime milkshakes, smoothies, snacks.
   - Try another stimulant and, if no improvement, consider a nonstimulant.
   - Try cyproheptadine (Periactin) 4 mg once or twice daily (antihistamine), which often stimulates appetite.
   - Supplement meals with instant breakfast drink, high-calorie bars, etc.
   - Rarely, consider half doses on weekends and holidays, or no medications in summer.
   - Consult a nutritionist.
3) Sleep problems (e.g., insomnia)
   - Establish good bedtime routine.
   - Give AM dose earlier.
   - Switch from 12- to 8-h medication.
   - Eliminate caffeine and energy drinks.
   - Try another stimulant. If symptoms persist, then try melatonin, 1–2 mg, at bedtime, occasionally may need 5–6 mg.

PEARL: There is a concern that melatonin can suppress other hormones, e.g., growth hormone, follicle stimulating hormone. There is no substantial or definitive evidence yet, but perhaps consider using smallest dose possible and stopping after 2–3 months, or using intermittently.
   - Consider a nonstimulant, e.g., atomoxetine, given once daily h.s. (at bedtime), or add an α-agonist, e.g., Intuniv, Kapvay, h.s.
   - Consider small doses of clonidine, e.g., 0.1–0.2 mg h.s. (generic short-acting α-agonist). Cheaper!
   - Rarely, in adolescents with symptoms of sleep deprivation consider giving trazodone.
   - Consider other coexisting problems, e.g., anxiety/depression, or consult a sleep specialist.

PEARL: R/O physical/sexual abuse.

4) Behavioral rebound (afternoon)
This occurs because of the sudden wear off of the stimulant effect in the afternoon and at end of school day.
   - Try longer sustained medications, e.g., 8–12 h.
   - Add a smaller dose in the afternoon on arriving home.
   - Overlap stimulant doses.
   - Try a different stimulant.
   - Last result change to nonstimulant.
   - Add a nonstimulant to the regimen, e.g., an α-agonist, in the morning.

5) Dizziness and syncope (rare)
   - Review cardiac history, symptoms, etc., in patient and family.
   - Monitor BP and pulse.
   - Ensure adequate fluid and calorie intake.
   - Consider change of medication, perhaps a nonstimulant such as atomoxetine.
   - Discontinue medications if adverse cardiac event occurs and consult a cardiologist. α-Agonists can cause postural hypotension.

6) Irritability (unusual)
   - Decrease dosage.
   - Try another stimulant or a different class of medication.
   - If chronic then consider other associated conditions, e.g., anxiety and/or depression, bipolar disorder, disruptive mood dysregulation disorder.

7) Exacerbation of tics
   - If the patient has preexistent tics prior to medication, stimulant medications may increase tics, decrease tics, or cause no change in tics.
   - Evaluate the effects of tic on the child, e.g., if noticeable (peers), bothersome, socially unacceptable, disruptive to class, injury to skin by chronic "picking at it." If so, it needs to be treated.
   - Reduce dosage.
   - Try a different stimulant.
   - Switch to a nonstimulant (atomoxetine has no effect on tics!).
   - Consider adding a long-acting α-agonist to the regimen.
   - Very unlikely that any treatment will totally eliminate the tics.

8) Hallucinations (very rare)
   - Stop treatment.
   - Consider trying a nonstimulant.

   - If symptoms persist then consult a child psychiatrist.

9) Psychosis (e.g., bug phobia), mania, depression, anxiety
   - Compare current with baseline assessment.
   - Stop stimulant if there is new onset or worsening of preexistent symptoms, e.g., mania, anxiety/depression.
   - In case of "bug phobia," fear to go outside because of fear of spiders, bees, etc. (proven side effect to stimulant medications) stop medications. Compare with baseline. If symptoms persist then refer to a child psychiatrist.
   - Try another medication, e.g., a nonstimulant.
   - Refer to a child psychiatrist.

10) "Zombiness"
   - Paradoxic oversedation due to excessive medication response.
   - Decrease dosage.
   - May need to change medications.

11) Weight loss (or height loss)
   - A 2-to 4-pound weight loss during early weeks of initiation is common. May be only partly regained.
   - Children and adolescents on stimulants usually thin out over time.
   - Monitor height often (e.g., every 3 months). If falling off previous height percentile, then lower the dose or discontinue medications and try a nonstimulant or increase calories (noted earlier).
   - If continues to fall off curve then do more growth assessment, e.g., to R/O thyroid, growth hormone, renal problems.

Side Effects of α-Agonists (Guanfacine, Clonidine, etc.)

1) Most common is sedation
   - Give medication twice daily or at bedtime only
2) Postural hypotension
   - Occurs more in adolescents
   - Usually tolerable; if not decrease dose or discontinue medication

Side Effects of Atomoxetine

1) Stomach discomfort, usually mild and temporary. If severe, or intolerable, discontinue medication.
2) Daytime drowsiness.
Start with PM dose only for 30 days and then go to AM dose. If symptoms persist, then try twice daily dosing or return to PM dosing only.

3) Jaundice
   - Baseline or periodic laboratory work (e.g., liver enzymes) not necessary.
   - Discontinue medications if jaundice occurs and do laboratory work (liver functions, etc.).
   - Monitor for persistence of symptoms.
   - Evaluate for other causes if symptoms persist.
   - If symptoms remit then try another class of medication.
4) Suicidal ideation
   - Stop treatment and screen for depression.
   - Consider referral to mental health.
5) Dizziness and syncope
   - Review family and child cardiac history and symptoms.
   - Monitor BP and pulse.
   - If persists then discontinue medications and consult pediatric cardiology.

Common Errors in Treatment
Overall errors

1) Treating only with medication, not using multi-modality therapy.
   - Parent/child education about ADHD
   - School interventions (IDEA, 504 plan, etc.)
   - Behavior therapy
   - Medications
2) Inadequate parent education on behavior modification techniques.
3) Using play therapy.
4) Not using rating scales (teacher and parent) to monitor response to therapy (i.e., medications).
5) Not increasing doses to the maximum, e.g., push to the maximum dose allowed or until side effects become intolerable.
6) Not assessing for coexistent conditions (anxiety, depression, learning problems, etc.).

Medication errors

1) Not proactively discussing possible side effects (e.g., decreased appetite) so that they can be dealt with promptly and noncompliance can be prevented.
2) Not monitoring growth properly (optimal every 3 months).
3) Giving up without adequate trial, e.g., may need to try two or three medications.
4) If school performance deteriorates then assess for medication compliance (may be spitting it out, etc.).
5) Switching medications because of potential self-limited side effects, e.g., stomach upset.
6) Not pushing medications to the maximum dosage.

PEARL: Risk factors for poor outcomes in ADHD.
1) Severity of ADHD, e.g., hyperactive/impulsive male with conduct disorder/aggressiveness. (high-risk child/adolescent)
2) Lower socioeconomic status/single parent/poor resources
3) Lower IQ
4) Maternal depression
5) Father is a substance abuser

Children in these situations should be monitored more closely. Unfortunately, the opposite, for obvious reasons, is often true.

Reference: ADHD: Clinical Practice Guideline for the Diagnosis, Evaluation, and Treatment of Attention-Deficit/Hyperactivity Disorder in Children and Adolescents. *Pediatrics* 128(5), November 2011.

ADHD MEDICATIONS: ASSESSMENT FOR CARDIAC RISK

Case Vignette: Parents of Eric, a 7-year-old second grader, come in for a summary visit, following an evaluation by you that resulted in a diagnosis of ADHD, combined type. The purpose of this visit includes the discussion of treatment options, including parent training in behavior therapy, school accommodations, and possibly a medication trial.

Both parents have done some online search on ADHD and express their concerns about sudden death (SD) that, their reading says, has occurred in children who take ADHD medications. They state that Eric has always been healthy, but their previous pediatrician stated that he has an "innocent heart murmur," which seems to "come and go." Also, the father's uncle "dropped over dead" at age 50 years with a heart attack. The parents feel "reluctant to consider ADHD medications unless a pediatric cardiologist is consulted."

Stimulant medications have been prescribed for patients with ADHD (literally millions of them) for more than 50 years, with a high level of comfort in using them. Is this comfort justified? Are there long-term safety consequences we have missed? Do we have adequate data to answer these questions? How should we decide who should or should not receive these medications, and how should we monitor them?

In 2005, the Pediatric Advisory Committee to the FDA decided to review possible adverse side effects and earlier reports regarding methylphenidate that surfaced that year. Two safety concerns were identified: psychiatric and cardiovascular adverse events. A call for more research data was made by the committee. Instead, the FDA Drug Safety and Risk Management Advisory Committee recommended a "black-box" warning of SD risk be placed on all prescriptions for stimulant medication. The FDA Pediatric Advisory Committee disagreed and ruled that a causal relationship between a stimulant medication and sudden cardiovascular death in a child with no cardiac anomaly was unproven. Instead, a recommendation was made to provide information to parents at the time of prescription to highlight potential risks, benefits, and possible side effects.

In reviewing data regarding SD in children, the FDA committee found that the incidence of SD in children was very low—about 0.6–6 per 100,000 (compared with the adult rate of SD of 1 per 1000 per year). The presumed cause of most SD cases in children was underlying congenital heart disease.

Data reviewed by the committee showed that from 1999 through 2003, there were 25 reports of SD in patients taking stimulants (7 children and 1 adult taking methylphenidate) and 17 patients (12 children and 5 adults) taking amphetamine. Risk-ratio rates of SD revealed adjusted rates of 0.16 for methylphenidate and 0.53 for amphetamine per 1 million prescriptions. (From the preceding two paragraphs, it is apparent that the risk of SD in patients taking stimulant medications was less than the overall risk of SD in the pediatric population.) Although these data do not totally rule out a cardiac risk in taking stimulant medications in childhood, they do show that if there is a risk, it is extremely low.

PEARL: More importantly, it is a much smaller risk to the child than growing up with untreated ADHD and all its potential negative possibilities (motor vehicle accidents, substance abuse, severe mental health issues, academic failure, etc.).

We know from research that the stimulant medications can affect vital signs, e.g., 2–4 mm Hg increase in systolic BP, 1–3 mm Hg increase in diastolic BP, and increase in heart rate from 3 to 5 beats per minute. These changes are statistically significant; however, they are not clinically significant.

No evidence of significant electrocardiographic (EKG) changes, e.g., in atrial or intraventricular conduction, had been noted, but theoretically a possible association with arrhythmias could be postulated.

Even though the possibility of underreporting was likely, the Pediatric Advisory Committee to the FDA believed that data in children were insufficient to assume a causal relationship between stimulant medications and sudden cardiac death. What the committee did emphasize, however, was the importance of screening children prior to the initiation of stimulant medications for possible signs or symptoms of cardiac disease (discussed later).

What about using stimulant medication in a child with a known structural abnormality of the heart? No one really knows the answer. Of the 19 deaths in children who were on stimulants, not all had autopsies or complete family or cardiac histories. Some of those 19 deaths did have structural abnormalities, but not all. Given that information, the decision to use stimulant medication in children with congenital heart disease will demand more intense screening and cardiac consultation (see later discussion) than in the child with a normal cardiac structure.

Despite all the data collection, risk determination, and thoughtful recommendations, the whole matter was reopened for debate when the American Heart Association, after thoughtful consideration, produced a report with a recommendation that an EKG be added to the cardiac and family history of risk factors, along with the PE, prior to initiation of stimulant medication. It was felt that this would identify conditions such as hypertrophic cardiomyopathy, long QT syndrome, and Wolff-Parkinson-White syndrome that are adverse conditions, making stimulant therapy more risky. The argument was that cardiac arrhythmias might not be identified by cardiac history and PE. They recognized, however, that there was no evidence base of data to substantiate this recommendation.

The American Academy of Pediatrics (AAP) subcommittee, upon review of the abovementioned report, disagreed with the AHA recommendation and issued a policy statement in May 2008 stating their dissent. They even went so far as stating that "harm outweighs the benefit" in following the AHA recommendation (e.g., cost to screen thousands of children, false-positive results, or other information that would interfere with the child from receiving optimal ADHD treatment, family anxiety, etc.). Again the AAP reviewed the 5-year data showing the risk of SD in stimulant-treated patients with ADHD to be not only miniscule but also less than the overall incidence of sudden cardiac death in the entire pediatric population.

The AAP (and the American Academy of Child and Adolescent Psychiatry) issued a joint statement recommending (summarized) the following:
1) **Careful assessment** prior to starting stimulant therapy using a "targeted cardiac history" (see later discussion).
2) For most children, primary care and specialty clinicians continue to provide the recommended treatment for ADHD, including stimulant medications, without obtaining routine EKGs or routine cardiac consultations. However, the final decision to

obtain an EKG was left to the discretion of the child's physician.

3) If there is a known history of cardiac disease or if a PE suggests possible cardiac disease, then evaluation by a cardiologist should be obtained.

Targeted Cardiac Screening
Child history (per parent)

1) Fainting and dizziness with exercise
2) Unusual shortness of breath with exercise
3) Chest pain with exercise
4) Decrease in exercise tolerance
5) Palpitations, missed heart beats
6) High BP
7) Heart murmur
8) Seizures
9) Heart surgery
10) Heart disease

Family history

1) Sudden, unexplained death at <50 years of age
2) "Heart attack" at <35 years of age
3) SD during exercise, or an event needing resuscitation
4) Cardiac arrhythmias
5) Cardiac myopathy (cardiac muscle disease)
6) Abnormal heart rhythm, e.g., long QT, short QT, Wolff-Parkinson-White syndrome
7) Sensorineural hearing loss
8) Marfan syndrome (or any syndromes)

PE

Height, weight, BP, pulse rate
Auscultate heart (rhythm, rate, murmur, etc.)

ADHD COACHING

Case Vignette: The parents and Stuart, their 17-year-old 10th grader, come to the clinic for a quarterly ADHD follow-up appointment. They are "exhausted," they say, trying to manage Stuart's ADHD. "It's a 24-h daily battle to get him to do what we ask."

For example, he refuses, or forgets, to do his homework on time, or does not even keep track of what he has to do or forgets to bring the right books home. They arranged a homework tutor, but he "forgets to go there." They arranged study skills classes at the local Sylvan agency, but he "forgets the appointment." Even when they help him all weekend on a major project, he "forgets to turn it in for several days," so his grade suffers.

They describe Stuart as a "nice boy." "Everybody loves him." But he is so "scattered" their relationship has turned into constant nagging. They even tried to increase his ADHD medication, but that did not help. So now he just "goes to his room and refuses to talk."

Teacher's progress reports state that his focus in class is "very good," and test scores show he is learning adequately, but his grades are suffering due to his failure to complete his homework in a timely fashion. Parents feel it is "more of a problem with organization and time management."

Both parents have "high-powered executive-type jobs." They summarize by jokingly saying "Stuart would do just fine if he had a personal secretary."

ADHD coaching is a concept that surfaced in the mid-1990s, although it had been utilized for many years in other arenas. No legal training or special certification is required to call oneself an ADHD coach, which results in two different vocational tracks to arrive at the title of "ADHD coach."

The first is to base one's expertise on life training, e.g., an adult with no specific coaching education but who has raised a difficult child with ADHD and has, along the way, learned a great deal about educational and behavioral issues surrounding ADHD. This then becomes the basis for marketing oneself as a "coach." Most persons who come along this track have skills in being a good listener, providing empathy and understanding, and giving advice based on their life experiences.

The other track to become an ADHD coach is to attend a coaching course in an approved training program. These are usually 2-year programs that provide certification and credentialing. One would presume such training would provide more skill and expertise than the first track. Often persons utilizing this track have previous training and credentialing in educational, nursing, and counseling fields.

A) What can ADHD coaches offer? The following points denote the myriad ways in which an ADHD coach offers help to the students with ADHD and their family:

1) They become "surrogate parents" in monitoring homework production and completion, meeting deadlines, and related roles that "burned-out" parents are struggling to provide.
2) They help the student plan and study for tests.
3) They help with realistic goal setting and how to achieve those goals.
4) They usually do not tutor but arrange tutoring in areas of academic weakness or deficiency.
5) The ADHD coach, by definition, understands the challenges of having ADHD, such as goal

setting, organization, prioritizing, time management, and all the aspects of executive function that are lacking or deficient in students with ADHD.

6) They help the child develop self-advocacy skills.

7) They can provide advocacy with the school to arrange for 504 plan accommodations.

8) They may represent the student, along with the parents, at school guidance team meetings.

9) They may, on occasion, provide transportation to needed resources, e.g., tutoring center.

10) They can provide help to the graduating child with ADHD regarding pursuit of college education vs. vocational training, including choices, application forms, etc.

B) What are the specific requirements of a coach?

1) They should possess skill and experience working with adolescents so that "bonding" and trust occur.

2) Their help should be personalized to the specific needs of the student.

3) They must get to know the student in a supportive role so that if or when insidious problems present, such as anxiety or depression, they are recognized early and treated promptly.

4) They must gain an understanding of family dynamics.

5) They should have good mediating, negotiating, and advocating skills and be readily available.

From all the abovementioned points, it is obvious that an ADHD coach should not only have experience or a thorough knowledge of the educational process but also have a thorough knowledge of ADHD and its symptom traits, impairments, and potential coexistent problems. Usually a background in nursing, education, psychology, or counseling best provides the prerequisite knowledge to prepare one for the vocation of ADHD coach.

Some excellent websites regarding ADHD coaching and superb books on the subject by outstanding authorities in the field are listed in the following.

C) Organizations/training programs

1) ADD Coach Academy (www.addcoachacademy.com)

2) ADHD Coaches Organization (www.adhdcoaches.org)

3) Institute for the Advancement of ADHD Coaching (www.adhdcoaches.org/circle/iaacadhd.coach-certification)

4) Professional Association of ADHD Coaches (www.paaccoaches.org

D) Resources (Books)

1) Nancy Ratey. *The Disorganized Mind: Coaching Your ADHD Brain to Take Control of Your Time, Tasks, and Talents.* New York: St. Martin's Press (2008).

2) P. Dawson and R. Guare. *Coaching Students with Executive Skills Deficits.* New York: Guilford Press (2013).

3) P. Quinn, N. Ratey, and T. Maitland. *Coaching College Students with ADHD: Issues and Answers.* Bethesda, MD: Advantage Books (2000).

4) J. Sleeper-Triplett. *Empowering Youth with ADHD: Your guide to coaching adolescents and young adults for coaches, parents, and professionals.* Plantation, FL: Specialty Press/A.D.D. Warehouse (2010).

E) Research

Field, Parker, Sawilowsky, and Rolands. *Quantifying the effectiveness of coaching for college students with ADHD.* Final Report to the Edge Foundation, Detroit (August 2010). Findings:

• students formulated more realistic goals,

• better time management,

• students felt less stressed, increased self-confidence, and more sense of empowerment.

ADHD ALTERNATIVE/COMPLEMENTARY TREATMENTS

Case Vignette: Mrs. Jones and her daughter Teresa, a 15-year-old ninth grader, whom you recently diagnosed with ADHD, inattentive type, come in to discuss treatment options. Mrs. Jones describes herself as a "naturalist." (Teresa "rolled" her eyes at that statement.) She feels Americans "take too many meds when they could get the same results with diet, exercise, and vitamin supplements." She even brought along a copy of a magazine, written by a physician she notes, that reinforces her opinion.

She has read that ADHD medications are "addictive" and she blames ADHD medications for her first husband's (Teresa's father, who had ADHD and took medications) alcohol addiction. She has also read that the medications "stunt your growth and make ADHD kids more likely to abuse street drugs." She is unwilling to expose Teresa to those risks when a "good fish oil supplement" could do the job just as well.

However, she does concur that Teresa's inattentiveness is a real concern that "needs to be dealt with."

The following list summarizes disproven or un-proven treatments for ADHD, some of which are even potentially harmful.

A. Disproven/unproven but probably safe
  1) Eye-muscle training
  2) Hypnosis
  3) Play therapy
B. Disproven/unproven and potentially harmful
  1) Chiropractic manipulation
  2) Megavitamins
  3) Herbal or nutritional supplements
  4) "Off-label" medications
    • are not FDA approved
    • have limited usefulness
    • have safety concerns
  3) Others
    • "Energy drinks"
    • "Brain enhancers"
  4) Elimination diets
C. Possibly helpful (safe) but limited research data
  1) Neurofeedback
  2) Omega-3
  3) Cogmed training (for executive functioning)
D. Remember, the proven treatment helps for ADHD
  1) Education of child/adolescent and parent about ADHD
  2) Classroom helps and accommodations
  3) Behavior therapy
  4) Specific FDA-approved medications

WHAT TO DO WHEN YOUR FAVORITE ADHD MEDICATION DOES NOT WORK
Case Scenarios

1. An 8-year-old boy diagnosed with combined type of ADHD and treated with Concerta. Now on 36-mg dose, with great control of ADHD symptoms at school and until bedtime. Vanderbilt rating scales normalized at both home and school. Parent still has issues getting him ready for school. Barely catches the bus because of his distractibility in the morning. Medication "doesn't kick in" for an hour or so.
Recommend: Try a small dose of methylphenidate upon waking (e.g., 5 mg) to "jump-start" his ADHD control. (Some parents awaken their child an hour or so early and give the short-acting medication and then let them go back to sleep until the normal waking time. This approach apparently can work very well.)
Risk: Won't eat breakfast; may need to feed earlier, then get ready for school.

2. A 7-year-old male with combined type ADHD and doing very well on Concerta, 27 mg, for 6 months. Linear growth following previous percentile, but weight fallen to lower percentile.
Recommend (try one or all):
  • Push calories—breakfast drinks and caloric snacks after school and bedtime.
  • Consider no medications, or half doses, on weekends and in summer.
  • Try Periactin, 4 mg, one to two times daily (an antihistamine that often increases appetite).
  • Consult a nutritionist.

3. Same as the previous case. Parents tried all above-mentioned recommendations; however, linear length is falling off toward a lower percentile.
Recommend (other options):
  • Mom tried some leftover 18 mg but teacher says, "ADHD out of control."
  • Discontinue Concerta and try another methylphenidate such as Focalin, which may have less appetite suppression (remember, it is twice as strong as methylphenidate in Concerta, Metadate, Ritalin, etc., so the Focalin dose is half the Concerta dose).
  • Add an alpha-agonist, e.g. long-acting Intuniv 1−2 mg. once or twice daily to the lower dose of 18 mg of Concerta, to see if that helps control the ADHD.
  • Discontinue stimulant therapy and start atomoxetine at 1.4 mg/kg per day. If ADHD not adequately controlled after 4−6 weeks, then add in small doses of methylphenidate, e.g., 5−10 mg once or twice daily.
  • If growth continues to fall off assess for growth failure.

4. A 9-year-old male with ADHD that is well controlled on Concerta, 54 mg, but has great difficulty falling asleep.
Options:
  • Review "sleep hygiene" principles.
  • Consider melatonin, 1−2 mg, 30 min before bedtime (see earlier note on melatonin).
  • Consider clonidine, 0.1or 0.2 mg, at bedtime (for sleep) (or Kapvay, long-acting form).
  • Consider adding guanfacine, 1−2 mg, at bedtime (or Intuniv, long-acting form).
  • Consider decreasing the dose of Concerta to 45 mg/d (18 mg plus 27 mg) so long as ADHD remains under control.
  • Consider changing to atomoxetine, 1.4 mg/kg per day, at bedtime and then adding in some stimulant medication in the morning if the

teacher rating scales do not verify adequate ADHD control at school.

- Consider an 8-h methylphenidate (e.g., Metadate CD, Ritalin LA) to replace 12-h Concerta.

5. A 16-year-old male who has been doing well for the past year or so on a Ritalin LA dose of 80 mg now complains of feeling like a "zombie" much of the time and wants to stop his medication.

Options (strongly suspect he is overmedicated):

- Try dropping the dose by 10–25%. If he does not feel better do more assessment, e.g., R/O depression.

PEARL: As adolescents with ADHD gain better control of their symptoms, and as the symptoms lessen over time, the dosage that was needed earlier has become excessive, causing feelings of lethargy. Avoid making the mistake that lethargy ("zombiness") requires a dose increase.

6. A 16-year-old female diagnosed with ADHD, inattentive type, who is bright and capable but is doing poorly in high school, is barely passing, refuses to study (too boring), and does not complete much homework. Emphatically states she "will not put any of that medicine in her body" (but she occasionally smokes pot with friends, she has confided privately to her physician). Parents are exasperated.

Options:

Use bribery, as threats rarely work. She seems motivated by money and new clothes. Offer her a dollar for each pill she takes for the next 3 months. It almost always works! NEED TO CLEAR THIS APPROACH WITH PARENTS FIRST.

After 3 months, the adolescent finds out that things are going better, parents are "off her back," and, not uncommonly, she will carry on with the medication even without parental financial incentive.

7. A 12-year-old male with inattentive ADHD, with a mild vocal tic (throat clearing). Family and patient desire medication therapy. Stimulant medication initiated. As the dosage is titrated upward, the tic becomes more noticeable, just when the ADHD symptoms were getting under control. Parents dropped the medication dosage to the previous level, but the ADHD symptoms became a problem.

Options:

- Add an α-agonist, for example, long-acting Intuniv (or Kapvay) at bedtime. This should lessen the tic symptom and may even add to the ADHD treatment so that the combination of the lower dose of stimulant is now effective due to the added α-agonist.

- If ADHD is not controlled, however, increase the stimulant dose until it controls ADHD. Hopefully, Intuniv will prevent the tic from worsening as the stimulant is increased.

- Instead stop the stimulant and start atomoxetine, which has no effect on tics.

8. A 12-year-old lad who is doing very well on his morning dose of Vyvanse, 40 mg. Mom is a single parent and leaves for work before the child awakens. High-school sibling is supposed to make sure he gets his medication, but frequently both she and the patient "forget."

Options:

- Perhaps a neighbor can drop by to remind the child to take medication.

- Have medicine (or some extra pills) available at school (locked up). RN to give.

9. You have recently evaluated and diagnosed a 9-year-old with ADHD and want to initiate medication. Father states he was "addicted" to amphetamines in college, which makes you reluctant to consider stimulant therapy.

Options:

- Have the medicine locked up and dispensed at school.

- Consider prescribing Vyvanse, which is nonaddicting, but a stimulant. Vyvanse has no effect if "snorted" because it must be ingested to become biologically active. However, it can be "abused" in the sense of being taken (swallowed) by a person who wants to "cram" for a test, so in that sense the abuse is a "diversion" from the person for whom it was prescribed.

- Consider prescribing atomoxetine (nonstimulant).

10. You have a high–school patient with ADHD who has been doing great on his stimulant medication. Mom calls in and says in the past month, things have "been spiraling downward." He is not studying or doing any homework, is failing tests, and seems "evasive" when questioned where he has been, or asked how things are going.

Options:

- Consider whether medication dose is still adequate due to recent growth spurt. May try increasing the dose weekly until either side effects occur or maximum dose per body weight is attained:

2 mg/kg per day for methylphenidate

1 mg/kg per day for amphetamines

- Consider whether the adolescent is compliant with taking medication. May be spitting it out later.
- *Recommend*: Observe him taking the medication, including swallowing.
- If maximum dose reached without seeing improvement then consider trying a different type of stimulant medication.
- Consider whether adolescent has been smoking pot regularly, or if there is other substance abuse.
- Consider whether adolescent has developed depression.

PEARL: If adolescent takes generic medication then inquire whether pharmacy has changed pharmaceuticals and new generic is not effective; it occasionally occurs. New generic may not be effective. May need brand-name medication if previously used generic is no longer available.

11. You have diagnosed a 13-year-old adolescent female with ADHD, inattentive type. She has about 6-month delays in her academic skills. She responded well to a medication trial, and both teachers and parents see her more attentive. After 3 months of medication therapy, teacher informs the parents that "things are improved, but she is still struggling."

   Options:
   - If not at maximum dose for size then increase medication dose.
   - Assess for possible anxiety/depression, which, if present, are not being treated.
   - Do a learning evaluation because lack of a better response to ADHD medication therapy may suggest an underlying learning disorder needing tutoring or other accommodations.

12. You begin an interview with parents regarding their child's possibility of having ADHD. As soon as they sit down, they inform you they are "against medications and under no consideration would they ever consider them, based on what they have heard and read online."

   You respond by saying that you "hear their feelings and desire" but suggest that there are other therapeutic options, so "let's proceed with the evaluation."

   After the assessment is completed, and you have confirmed their child truly does have ADHD, they again state "no medications."

   You then discuss the multimodality treatment of ADHD:

   a) Parent/child education about the disorder, for example, books, websites, CHADD organization, etc. (see the list on Resources).

   b) School accommodations as needed, such as the 504 plan, special education/individualized educational plan, and tutoring.
   c) Behavior therapy.
   d) Medications.
   You gently suggest you concur with them, not to "prescribe medications," but encourage them to enroll in the parenting class to learn thoroughly on how to do behavior therapy.

PEARL: Within 3–4 weeks the parents return to request a medication trial.

   Why the change?
   They heard from other parents about the usefulness as well as the absence of significant side effects of medications.
   Without question, this is the best fallout from having a true (not virtual) parenting class—the interaction and reassurance from other parents.

NEUROFEEDBACK TREATMENT FOR ADHD

Important: First a word about what it takes to become a truly evidence-based treatment for ADHD. The FDA requires at least two multisite randomized controlled studies and two extended open-label safety efficacy studies. Very few nonmedication treatments come even close to meeting those requirements.

Neurofeedback is a treatment form that has been around for many years but has not been recommended by the AAP as an evidence-based treatment for ADHD because most studies suggesting its worth are flawed by bias sampling, inadequate number of cases, or other methodology issues. In addition, the cost of this treatment form is quite expensive, ranging from $3000 to $4000 for the 30 or so sessions. Although it is probably a safe treatment, it seems inappropriate to use that much amount of resource (vs. tutoring). The treatment involves using electroencephalography to train the patient to develop positive brain waves, e.g., focusing ones, rather than the negative ones causing inattention.

It is becoming more widely used by mental health professionals despite the denunciation by many experts in the ADHD field describing it basically as "quackery."

A school-based study in the Journal of Developmental Behavioral Pediatrics, January 2014, by N. Steiner et al. shows some evidence that this modality of treatment might offer some positive benefit.

PEARL: At this point, until more definitive double-blinded studies are available, it is perhaps more appropriate that we take a "wait-and-see" approach before advising parents to consider this quite expensive treatment form. It is probably better to use their financial resources elsewhere.

OMEGA-3 FOR ADHD TREATMENT

See earlier discussion on the requirements for FDA approval of ADHD treatments.

Omega-3 has been touted for several years as being helpful in treating several mental health conditions including anxiety, depression, and ADHD. The evidence for ADHD treatment has been rather weak. It is not approved treatment per the FDA.

The following review article, along with my comments, summarizes I believe current thinking.

M. Bloch, MD, and A. Qawasmi, MD. Omega-3 Fatty Acid Supplementation for the Treatment of Children with ADHD Symptomatology: Systematic Review and Meta-Analysis. *J Am Acad Child Adolesc Psychiatry* 50(10):991–1000, 2011.

Meta-analysis of 10 trials, including 699 children. The outcome measure was the mean difference in rating scales measuring the symptoms of ADHD severity, before and after treatment.

Results: "Omega-3 fatty acid supplementation demonstrated a small but significant effect in improving ADHD symptoms."

Comment: Certainly, this study does not support replacing stimulants or atomoxetine as the first-line treatment for ADHD, or even α-agonists as the second-line treatment. At best, it might be considered as an adjuvant treatment or may be given to children whose parents adamantly refuse giving evidence-based medications.

PEARL: What we found in our clinic, however, was that almost all parents, who attended an ADHD parent group, eventually agreed to a trial of stimulant medications. This decision undoubtedly was motivated by their speaking with fellow parents, whose child was on medication, whom they trusted perhaps more than us initially, as well as hearing about not only the significant positive effects but also the safety and relatively minimal side effects.

CHAPTER 5

Age and Gender Differences in ADHD Presentation

ADHD PRESCHOOL
Case Vignette

A mother brings her 4.5-year-old son to you because of uncontrolled behavior. He was just expelled from his fourth preschool because he would not sit down in circle time but cruised around the room making disruptive noises.

Mom is a single parent, living alone with grandma, who is the daytime babysitter. Dad, who left the family before the child's birth, is a fisherman who dropped out of high school and joined the Navy.

This was the mom's only pregnancy, which was unremarkable except the baby "kicked her all the time." His overall health and development otherwise seems normal.

Diagnosis and Treatment of ADHD in Preschool Children

Diagnosis and treatment of ADHD in preschool children can be very challenging, even to the clinician who is very experienced in this disorder. Why?

1. The symptoms attributed as ADHD traits may be normal developmental traits for this age child. (Remember, "all 2-year-old children fulfill the ADHD criteria!" And some children are slower in "outgrowing" these normal developmental traits.)
2. Often, observations are not from two environments (e.g., school and home) but information only from home. If home is a chaotic environment, this information may be misleading. Similarly, information from a daycare/preschool environment that is unstructured, or from observers who are not trained or sophisticated, can also be misleading.
3. Medication response does not prove the diagnosis (at this age or any age).
4. Methylphenidate (MPH) is the only medication that has been studied in a randomized controlled trial in preschool-aged children. It is more potent and produces side effects at lower doses in this age group. The side effects in preschool-aged children are the same as in older children but they occur more often

and may be more prominent. Hence the need to start with a very small initial dose and proceed slowly.

5. In preschool-aged children limit medication treatment of ADHD to those with moderate to severe symptoms and/or aggression.
6. Follow the American Academy of Pediatrics Guidelines for preschool ADHD diagnosis and treatment (Pediatrics, November 2011).

"First try behavioral interventions, such as group or individual parent training in behavior management techniques." (Note: What is meant is an intensive group or 1:1 parenting instruction over several sessions, not just attending a simple "parenting class.")

There are two reasons for this intensive approach. First, it may be clear through direct observations whether the behavioral issues are due to ADHD or inappropriate parenting. Second, if ADHD seems to be the apparent diagnosis, the parents have learned to do the behavior therapy component of ADHD treatment. See Resources chapter 18 FOR LIST OF BEHAVIOR PROGRAMS FOR PARENTS OF PRESCHOOL CHILDREN.

- MPH may be considered when there is no significant improvement (lessening) of behavior symptoms.
- Start with a low dose of MPH, e.g., 2.5 mg bid.

7. Use only short-acting MPH (never start with long-acting medications in preschool-aged children) and titrate up to 7.5 mg tid.
8. If intensive behavior therapy is not feasible or available, then consider the risks versus benefits of a medication trial.
9. Monitor frequently, e.g., weekly visits for the first month, to observe for side effects, including emotional lability, decreased appetite, sleep problems, weight loss, or growth decline. Continue this and then schedule return visits at 2 weeks for four to eight visits until stable on medications with no significant side effects. Then see monthly.

PEARL: Medications in preschool children are effective at lower doses and are more likely to cause side effects.

A definitive study of ADHD in preschool children by Greenhill et al. is the Preschool ADHD Treatment Study (PATS) that was published in the *Journal of the American Academy of Child and Adolescent Psychiatry* in November 2006.

Results: PATS

Short-acting MPH, at doses of 2.5, 5, and 7.5 mg, produced significant reductions in symptom scales in preschoolers compared with school-aged children on the same medication.

- Treatment was initiated at the lowest dose (2.5 mg bid).
- Effective size of dosage was smaller than that in school-aged children.
- Start with 2.5 mg bid and increase to 2.5 mg tid after 1 week.
- Mean daily dose, 14.1 mg +/− 8.1 mg/day.
- Higher rates of emotional lability noted than school-aged children.
- Higher incidence of adverse side effects, e.g., appetite, weight, growth.

PEARL: MPH is an effective treatment for preschool children with ADHD, but at lower doses, with increased side effects compared with their school-aged counterparts.

PEARL: The CDC Morbidity and Mortality Weekly Report dated April 5, 2016, showed that in preschool ADHD-diagnosed children, only 50% received behavior therapy, but 75% were given medications.

In preschool ADHD, behavior therapy should be the first option. It may even help confirm the ADHD diagnosis, which in preschool children can be challenging.

ADHD IN ADOLESCENTS: DIAGNOSTIC AND THERAPEUTIC PITFALLS

Case Vignette: Alec is a 16-year-old high-school sophomore, who was diagnosed with ADHD, combined type, in elementary school. He subsequently did well on ADHD medications and behavior therapy (which parents received from a parenting class offered at their medical facility). Because he struggled academically in the early school years, an individualized educational plan evaluation was done, which demonstrated a specific learning disability in reading and math.

He received special education for 4 years and eventually was felt to be at grade level academically, so it was discontinued. Writing, however, still remains a challenge.

"Things have gone South this year" the parents say. They smell smoke on his clothes and have concerns that he is also smoking pot. He has been arrested twice for speeding, and currently, his license to drive is on "hold." His school work has deteriorated, with many incompletes. Parents have hired a homework tutor. He is barely passing his grades due to missing or late assignments. If things do not improve, school says, "he will have to go to Summer school."

Parents wonder if his medication has "lost its effect." Now he objects to taking it because his friends "don't like him when he takes his medications."

As described in the introductory chapter 3 on ADHD, the symptoms present differently depending on the developmental age of the patient, e.g., preschoolers and early school children present mostly with overactivity and impulsive behavior, whereas in adult life the issues are more significant in the areas of relationships (family, society, and job) and executive function.

Adolescence presents some challenges in both diagnosis and treatment, not only because of the unique problems of that developmental age but also in how ADHD presents in males versus females. These challenges, and some tips for meeting those challenges, are listed in the following.

A) ADHD in adolescent males (not all traits seen in every adolescent)
   1) Usually the combined type of ADHD.
   2) More likely to have been diagnosed early in first grade if not preschool because they are usually disruptive, hard to control in a larger class size, and may get removed from the classroom and be sent for an assessment.
   3) The hyperactivity is motoric, easily noted.
   4) May "act out," be aggressive and antisocial.
   5) Poor social skills, often few friends, and rare social invites.
   6) Tendency to deny problems and blame others ("teacher is stupid").
   7) All these issues persist from childhood into adolescence, causing lack of self-esteem, poor school performance, and the slow downward spiral of academic performance, even without the presence of a coexisting learning disorder.
   8) Oppositional defiant disorder is a common coexistent problem (∼50%): ignores or defies rules.

9) Conduct disorder is common ($\sim$20%): fighting, bullying, breaking into and entering, stealing, etc.

10) Frequent driving issues: traffic violations, accidents.

11) Substance abuse: tobacco, alcohol, cannabis.

12) Teacher rating scales often not helpful in assessment process because of the teacher's lack of knowledge about the child's classroom behavior (large number of pupils, multiple teachers).

13) Poor executive function: poor homework and project completion, or delay in turning it in.

14) Lots of failed grades due to incomplete work; need to repeat class in summer school.

15) Often poor or weak athletic skills due to weak gross motor function. Not competitive in athletics (however, there are exceptions, e.g., Michael Phelps).

16) So adolescent males with ADHD often fail in three major domains: friends, school, and sports. No wonder they act out their anger!

PEARL: The abovementioned describes about two-thirds of adolescent boys with ADHD. About one-third are the inattentive type and present with symptoms more like the typical ADHD adolescent female.

Case Vignette: Carolyn is a 14-year-old high-school freshman who comes in with her parents who wonder if she might have ADHD (actually, the school counselor advised them to seek medical help). Parents describe Carolyn as a delightful young child who was "always happy and exuberant, though overly talkative at times." School has by and large gone well mostly because she is so well liked by her peers and teachers. She uses her family to help her complete assignments, or gets a "pass" from the teacher, as she is quite bright, and school seems to come easily. The parents' current concerns regard her "out of character" behavior, e.g., she has been caught shoplifting on two occasions and her mom found a pack of cigarettes in her coat pocket. Her school performance has declined recently due to late or missing assignments.

B) ADHD in adolescent females
1) Hyperactivity is often mostly verbal ("chatty Cathy") or just "fidgety."
2) They are more likeable, less obnoxious, and rarely aggressive.
3) As they are usually not hyperactive or obnoxious and not a class behavior problem or disruptive, they often escape diagnostic consideration until middle school or high school.
4) What happens then is that they are finally held accountable for work completion, which they are not very good at doing, but in early school years, they were not held accountable.
5) This delay in diagnosis is also often facilitated by parents who "enable them," e.g., excessive help with homework completion
6) If they do not have enabling parents or teachers, they surface as problems much earlier.
7) The concomitant presence of a learning disorder coexisting with ADHD also aids in earlier recognition of problems.
8) Usually poor executive function: messy work, often forgetful, poor work completion, procrastinates, but gets a "pass" in early years because of their likeability.
9) Teacher rating scales may be invalid due to lack of overt behavioral symptoms.
10) Usually social skills are okay, so has a group of friends (who also might "cover" for them). However, often less attentive to "social cues."
11) Tendency "to internalize," e.g., school failure, peer rejection, so more likely to develop anxiety/depression than acting out behavior.
12) Lack of self-esteem is common.

C) Diagnostic recommendations (for both male and female patients with ADHD)
1) **PEARL:** Review all school report cards since kindergarten/first grade. ADHD does not just "show up in the seventh or eighth grade." There is usually a paper trail in the teacher comments suggesting issues of inattention, need for prodding, one-to-one help, etc. Progress reports may be more helpful than grades per se.
2) Remember that one-third or so of males with ADHD fit the inattentive type category and one-third or so of females fit the combined type (with hyperactivity).
3) The 1:1 interview is especially crucial for the evaluation of ADHD in adolescence (see previous chapter 3 regarding what interview entails).
4) Adolescent to complete an ADHD self-report (see Chapter 1)
5) **PEARL:** Always screen for coexistent conditions such as anxiety and depression, as they may either mimic ADHD symptoms, and be

the primary diagnosis, or accompany ADHD as a coexistent problem (use specific ratings scales per chapters 9 on anxiety and 12 on depression).

6) Consider academic testing if the adolescent complains of school being "hard" or if there are academic delays, even if the adolescent has not needed or received special education (he/she may have fallen through the cracks because his/her deficiencies were "not bad enough").

7) Always consider substance abuse testing, as substance abuse commonly occurs in adolescents with ADHD and certainly causes inattention and school deterioration.

8) Do not rely totally on rating scales for ADHD, for the reasons noted earlier. Negative rating scales do not rule out ADHD!

9) Consider calling the school counselor because that person might have important and helpful information (regarding the adolescent and his or her issues, family, peers, social skills, etc.).

10) **PEARL:** Remember, adolescents with ADHD tend to be immature for their age and peers (possibly 2–3 years). This explains some of their lack of motivation to succeed.

D) Therapeutic recommendations for both male and female patients with ADHD

1) The biggest challenge is getting the homework done and turned in.

2) Consider a 504 plan (a "must" in my book for most, if not all, adolescents with ADHD). It includes
- modifying assignments (shortened?);
- providing grace period, e.g., 24–48 h for homework, 5 days for projects (as homework is often not turned in on time even if completed);
- arranging a study skills class;
- "homework club" after school, if available;
- hiring a "homework tutor" (even an older peer) to assist with and facilitate homework completion;
- hiring an "ADHD coach" (see section re: ADHD Coach in chapter 4).

For more information see chapter on 504 Plan.

3) Medication issues: If ADHD symptoms worsen, or school deteriorates, consider the following:
- May need a dose adjustment, or different medication.

- Noncompliance in taking medication, e.g., "spits out later"—monitor swallowing (peer pressure against medications).
- Diversion? Keep medicine locked up.
- Onset of substance abuse, such as cannabis.
- New coexistent problems such as anxiety/depression—see clinician, do screening, etc.
- Refuses to take medicines then
    negotiate monthly (or twice to thrice) with rewards,
    BRIBE, e.g., $1.00 for each pill taken (if parents agree).

4) Self-esteem, social issues—consider summer camps, wilderness experience.

Reference: Wolraich ML, et al. Attention-deficit/hyperactivity disorder among adolescents: a review of the diagnosis, treatment, and clinical implications. *Pediatrics.* 2015;115(6).

ADHD GOES TO COLLEGE

Case Vignette: Robert and his parents have made an appointment to discuss college options. He is just starting his senior year in high school and has done quite well, considering the diagnosis of ADHD, inattentive type, for which he still takes ADHD medications. His vocational dream is to become a civil engineer like his father.

Dad would like him to attend his own alma mater, a small private college in Ohio, about a day's drive away. Mom is unsure whether he is even ready to go to college. She admits he still needs her to "keep him organized," e.g., getting his assignments and projects in on time and remembering when major tests are scheduled.

Both agree he "might not be ready to go away to college at this time" and wonder what other options are available.

Entry to college presents some unique challenges to an adolescent with ADHD. Fortunately, there are many available tools and resources at the adolescent's disposal to lessen the stress and assure the likelihood of success. The three key ingredients to a rewarding and successful college experience are PLAN, PLAN, and PLAN!

The following thoughts, in a question format, outline what factors must be taken into account in deciding the What, How, When, and Where questions regarding attending college.

A) How does ADHD impact learning (and thus affect the success of the educational process at any level)? In addition to its core symptoms (overactivity, inattention, and impulsivity), ADHD has a major negative impact on executive function, including skills such as

1) organization,
2) time management (including procrastination),
3) working memory,
4) neatness and orderliness,
5) consistency and productivity,
6) study skills,
7) ability to work independently.

PEARL: Some research suggest that executive function skills are more important factors than academic skill deficits (e.g., in math, writing) in determining the success or failure of the college experience. It is crucial that the college-bound adolescent has mastered these skills to the fullest extent possible (discussed more later).

B) Am I ready for college (e.g., in terms of emotional maturity, independence, self-starting, self-regulation)? Children with ADHD mature less rapidly than their peers. They might not be ready to function independently at 18 years of age. How do we prepare them to go off to college? Consider the following options:

1) Stay at home for a year or two and attend a community college.
2) Learn some self-management skills such as public transportation, time and money management, laundry, meal preparation, social life, exercise routines (necessary for parent to "pull away" and foster these skills development).
3) Use this time to complete the basic "core" courses most colleges require.
4) Optionally take some vocational courses. Many vocations, such as automechanics, bookkeeping, medical assistant, and 20–30 others, can be completed in a 2-year educational program, yielding a certificate or associate degree and an availability for employment. Many adolescents with ADHD prefer a "hands-on" type of vocation.
5) Many adolescents with ADHD profit a great deal from the abovementioned approach. It provides just a little more time to grow up.
6) Have a part-time job to pay for their own personal expenses.

C) How do I choose a college? There are several important factors to keep in mind:

1) Distance from home, tuition expense, private versus public, availability of certain majors (e.g., nursing, education, engineering).

2) Small college versus large university. Smaller colleges, smaller class size, and more personal contact with instructors may be less intimidating to students with ADHD.
3) Availability of mentoring or tutoring. Schools with "learning centers" are more capable of providing the one-to-one help that students with ADHD need than larger schools without such a resource. These resources are often found in schools that have a Department of Education, i.e., the school is training teachers. The learning center would probably have personnel available to the student with ADHD or learning disability for mentoring and coaching.

Option: Hire a private tutor/coach to help the student with organization, time management, study skills, etc. It can be very helpful!

4) While choosing a college, it is very important for a student with ADHD to know in advance whether the college can provide these one-to-one resources. This information is usually available on the school's website or during the interview/visitation process.

D) What are my educational rights?

Adolescent students with ADHD who have had a 504 plan accommodation in high school can have that transferred to all public institutions of higher learning. It can provide many accommodations:

1) Extra time for tests (even SAT tests can be given with extra time if certain qualifications are presented).
2) Use of a notetaker, or a tape recorder.
3) Possibly tutoring.

E) How will my medication refills be handled?

Issues regarding medications need to be determined prior to the student's leaving for college. Questions include the following:

1) How will refills be given? All colleges have Student Health Services, but they may not refill ADHD medication.
2) Another dilemma is that the college may be in another state where the personal physician is not licensed.
3) Most ADHD medications are controlled substances and cannot be automatically refilled.
4) **PEARL:** It is important to remember that medication dosages and schedules will probably have to be altered after the student arrives at college because of the changing schedules and lifestyles. How will this be facilitated, e.g., student-to-physician contact?

5) **PEARL**: The most important point regarding all the abovementioned is that all these concerns need to be determined before the student departs to college.
6) Discuss diversion of medications (sale, giving away, etc.).

F) What other resources would be helpful to prepare the adolescent with ADHD for college?
This is where the primary care clinician can be very helpful in providing books and other resources.

1) **PEARL**: Book for students with ADHD Kathleen G. Nadeau, PhD. Survival Guide for College Students with ADHD or LD.
2) Book for parents of children with ADHD: Chris Dendy, M.S. Teenagers with ADD and ADHD. Read chapter on College.
3) Websites:
Children and Adults with Attention-Deficit/Hyperactivity Disorder (CHADD) organization, www.chadd.org
National Resource Center, www.help4adhd.org
Section 504 accommodations, www.ed.gov/ocr/
Coaching, www.edgefoundation.org
4) Consider electronic options such as phone apps to facilitate time management and organizational skills.
5) Consider audio books rather than reading from textbooks.
6) Take a study skills class (either in high school or in the local community college prior to entering college.
7) Prior to leaving for college:
   • Develop a crisis management plan when the student "hits a brick wall:"
     a) Whom to call at college (tutor, counselor, etc.)?
     b) Call home!

Resource: The Family Educational Rights and Privacy Act allows the parents to receive progress reports from their child's college, as long as the student signs a waiver of rights. This is helpful in monitoring the student's progress.
Resource: CHADD, National Resource Center, **www.help4adhd.org**. It has many good information regarding
1) finding the right college,
2) college and ADHD,
3) succeeding in college with ADHD,
4) disclosing ADHD during the college admissions process.

Resource: Peterson. Colleges with Programs for Students with LD or ADHD. 6th Edition. www.petersons.com; Marybeth Kravets and Imy F. Wax. The K&W Guide to Colleges for Students With Learning Disabilities or Attention Deficit Disorder.

ADULT ADHD
Case Vignette
John comes into the clinic at the insistence of his wife, Mary, who expressed an ultimatum that "if you don't go and get help, I'm leaving." John reluctantly came in because this was his third marriage and he "wanted to save it." What prompted this threat was John's recent firing when he showed up for work with alcohol on his breath.

John has had a very troubled history. His dad left when John was a teenager. John hated school, though he had been diagnosed with ADHD early on, and had taken medications, which helped. However, when he became a teenager, he stopped his medications because they "made him feel like a zombie." He dropped out of school when he was 16 years, but eventually got his General Educational Diploma (GED). Although he hated school, everyone who knows him says he is "smart."

He has had great trouble, he says, keeping a job because of "stupid bosses" who annoy him, so he "tells them off."

He drinks several cans of beer in the evening and smokes excessively, both of which "help him relax."

His relatives have told him he was "just like his dad."

ADHD in Adults
Adult ADHD was not formally considered a "disorder" until the 1980s. (However, Paul Wender, MD, adult psychiatrist, had been writing about the topic of adult attention deficit disorder [ADD].) Actually the diagnosis of ADHD was not often given to females because decades ago the emphasis was on "hyperactivity" and the term most commonly used for this problem was "the hyperactive child," a term almost exclusively applied to boys.

But in the 1980s the focus changed from the symptom of hyperactivity to inattention, and the advent of the term ADD was noted. As there were two types of ADD, one with hyperactivity and one without hyperactivity, lumping them together as ADHD was the next logical step. But, of course, this became an oxymoron because we needed two subtypes of ADHD, the inattentive type (no hyperactivity, usually the girls) and the combined type (hyperactive/impulsive as well as inattentive, usually the boys).

We used to tell parents that the child's condition would be "outgrown" by early adolescence because the hyperactivity would "go away." How wrong we were! It is true that the hyperactivity does usually lessen considerably, and perhaps even some of the impulsivity as well. But the inattentiveness persists often into young adult life or throughout adult life, and it is hard to say in truth whether the symptom is truly "improved" or whether getting out of school and into an interesting motivating vocation is what really lessens the symptoms, along with the individual's improved coping skills learned along the way.

Be all that as it may, we know now, with an extensive evidence base, that the symptoms (and impairment) from ADHD in childhood are still recognized in perhaps 50% or so of adults who grew up having an ADHD diagnosis. This translates into about 8–10 million American adults, men and women, who still carry this diagnosis or are living with impairments or coexistent conditions that developed as a result of ADHD. This is particularly true of those adults whose ADHD was either not recognized or recognized but not treated.

A) The symptoms in adult life of persistent ADHD are not that different from the symptoms of childhood/adolescence and includes
1) problems with relationships
2) smoking/alcohol/substance abuse
3) restlessness, inability to relax
4) procrastination
5) easily distracted
6) loses things a lot
7) disorganized
8) problems completing tasks
9) trouble on the job
10) quick temper
11) impulsive
12) thrill seeking

B) These ADHD symptom traits become increasingly impairing in adult life because of the complexities and high demands expected of an adult. So the result is that the person struggles, at times significantly, in one or more domains of life:
1) Educational: Attainment less than expected
2) Social: Lack of friends, isolation
3) Vocational: Conflicts with supervisors
4) Legal: Conflicts with law (e.g., drinking and driving)
5) Marital: Domestic violence, divorce
6) Financial: Debts, poor money management
7) Medical: Motor vehicle or other accidents, risk taking

C) A current thought about adult ADHD is that it did not "begin" in adulthood but was either not recognized as ADHD, or diagnosed, or misdiagnosed as something else, e.g., anxiety. There are several possible scenarios to illustrate how adult ADHD might be eventually diagnosed:
1) Child diagnosed with ADHD in childhood, continued medication through college, tried being off medications, realized he "needed" them, so has continued medications into adult life.
2) Child had symptoms that were milder, though noted, but had excellent parenting, school structure, and accommodations, with no apparent learning problems, and did well until adult life and was forced to function independently.
3) Adult has child diagnosed with ADHD. During the child's evaluation and treatment, parent realizes he (or she) had same issues as a child, still has some ADHD issues, gets diagnosed and treated.

PEARL: About 40%–50% of parents of children with ADHD had/still have ADHD symptom traits. Many still have issues. One of our roles, as we work with the child with ADHD, is to identify a parent with possible ADHD and facilitate an evaluation.
4) Adults seek counseling because of life issues:
- Spouse urged them, problems in marriage (see earlier case vignette)
- Recent job loss due to alcohol, conflict with boss, poor work performance, absenteeism, etc.
- Depressed adult due to "underachievement," "demoralization," "lost opportunities"
- Social consequences: Loss of driver's license due to alcohol
- Recent divorce
- Feeling they are a "failure"
5) Adults will often say "I've always known something is wrong, but I never knew what." They often feel relieved when the diagnosis is made.

D) Diagnosis of adult ADHD
1) Patient to complete the ADHD Adult Self-Report Scale (see Chapter 1)
2) Physical examination
- Rule out chronic illness (hypertension, diabetes, sleep apnea, anemia, thyroid, etc.)
3) Laboratory screening (as indicated)
- For above mentioned conditions
- Toxicology
- Sleep study
4) Screen for other mental health conditions, e.g., anxiety, depression.

E) Differential diagnosis
  1) Chronic medical condition
  2) Other mental health condition, e.g., anxiety/depression (primary vs. secondary diagnosis)
  3) Sleep apnea
F) Treatment
  1) Psychiatric consultation
  2) Counseling
     • Interpersonal versus cognitive behavior therapy
     • Marital
     • Vocational
  3) Substance abuse (alcohol, etc.) treatment
  4) Remedial education
  5) Vocational training
  6) Support group (CHADD, Alcoholics Anonymous, etc.)
  7) Medications
     • ADHD (stimulants, nonstimulants)
     • selective serotonin reuptake inhibitors (anxiety/depression, etc.)
     • Others

New-Onset ADHD in Adults: Is it for Real?

In the section ADHD in Adults, it was noted that ADHD in adults was a continuation of ADHD in childhood, and if it was not diagnosed until adulthood, it was because it was either missed; for example, because it was mild and compensated for by accommodations such as parent help, school interventions or it was called something else, such as an anxiety disorder or learning problem.

There has been an active discussion regarding "adult-onset ADHD," presuming that the disorder does not really present in some people until adulthood. An article in *JAMA Psychiatry*, July 2016, discusses that possibility.

For more information regarding this topic read the article by Goodman, et al. Diagnosis and treatment of ADHD in older adults: a review of the evidence and its implications for clinical care. *Drugs Aging*, January 2016.

CHAPTER 6

ADHD Transitioning to Adulthood

MAYA KUMAR, MD, FAAP

CASE VIGNETTE

Jamie is a 16-year-old male adolescent with combined-type ADHD diagnosed at 8 years of age. He initially had a great response to a combination of stimulant medication, behavior modification, and comprehensive individualized education plan (IEP) at school, getting straight *A*'s throughout middle school. But after starting high school, his grades dropped to a B average, which has really disappointed him and his parents. He only remembers to take his morning medication about half the time because he is in a rush to get to school and says "my mom forgets to remind me." He finds that his high-school IEP includes less one-on-one help than it did in middle school. His middle-school teachers used to do "binder checks" and prompted him to write things in his daily planner, but now "they expect me to do that stuff on my own." His mom is frustrated with him for not being more independent with doing his school work and taking care of himself. "I still wake him up for school every morning. Getting him off his phone to do his homework is a challenge. He doesn't even eat on his own unless I make something for him."

Jamie is worried about the future and whether he will get into a good college. "All my friends seem to have plans, but I'm not sure what I really want to do yet." His mom is worried about whether he will be ready for college, "He still seems so young." Confidentially Jamie discloses he occasionally uses alcohol and marijuana with his friends, and sometimes he uses marijuana when he is alone to relax when he feels stressed. Sometimes he takes an extra dose of his long-acting medication at night, so he can stay up late to finish his homework.

How can we help Jamie prepare for adulthood and an adult model of healthcare?

ADHD is often considered a childhood illness, and it is commonly believed that ADHD is usually outgrown by adulthood. However, about 75% of children diagnosed with ADHD continue to have elevated ADHD symptoms in young adulthood, with 60%

experiencing functional impairment.[1] Overall, about 4%–5% of adults have ADHD.[2] While there is some attenuation in ADHD symptoms with age and maturity, particularly impulsivity and hyperactivity, discontinuation rates of ADHD treatment in young adulthood are disproportionately higher. One large study of adolescents taking ADHD medication at age 16 years found that only 63% remained on medication by their 17th birthdays and only 41% remained on medication by their 18th birthdays.[3] Another study found that once they become college freshman, young people with ADHD only take about 37% of their medication doses.[4]

Children with ADHD often have many supports, including parents, pediatric healthcare providers, and educators, to help them manage their condition with pharmacologic and nonpharmacologic treatment. But as they grow up, they are expected to function more independently in their education, vocational pursuits, activities of daily living, and medical self-management. Regardless of a young adult's underlying condition, transitioning from a pediatric to an adult model of healthcare is a challenge. Some of the differences between these models are summarized in Table 6.1. When it comes to ADHD specifically, young adults may be doubly disadvantaged because of the nature of their condition. Failure to adhere to their treatment plans results in worsening of inattention and impulsivity, which further decreases their capacity to manage their health and perpetuates a vicious cycle.

Pediatric providers are often well versed in the consequences of poorly managed ADHD in childhood and adolescence, including poor academic performance, low self-esteem, difficulty with peer interactions, getting in trouble at school, and ill-advised experimentation with substances and sex. Unfortunately, the stakes get higher in adulthood and people have much more to lose from poorly managed ADHD. In adulthood, poorly controlled ADHD reduces overall educational attainment and employment,

TABLE 6.1
Differences Between Pediatric and Adult Healthcare Models

	Pediatric Healthcare	Adult Healthcare
Parental involvement	Encouraged	Discouraged
Health decision-making and consent	Parental	Individual
Access to health information	Parental	Individual
Availability of treatment providers	Well-established teams, often multidisciplinary, for pediatric conditions	Fewer providers for conditions starting in childhood
Healthcare logistics, including - identifying providers - booking appointments - transportation to appointments	Parental	Individual
Medication management, including - remembering to take medication - obtaining prescriptions - requesting refills on time	Parental	Individual
Financial support, including - insurance coverage - out-of-pocket costs (e.g., co-pays)	Parental	Individual is ultimately responsible; variable parental ability or willingness to assist

resulting in greater financial burden and reduced productivity that affects our society as a whole. Adults with uncontrolled ADHD are more likely to make errors while driving and are more likely to die from accidents. Consequences from impulsive sexual risk-taking and substance abuse become increasingly severe. The criminal justice system becomes less willing to forgive impulsive acts. Uncontrolled ADHD precludes the ability to adhere to treatment plans for other medical conditions, resulting in poorer overall physical health. Effects on social functioning become more profound, with fewer meaningful friendships and relationships and a higher rate of divorce. In other words, failing to prepare adolescents to manage their ADHD independently in adulthood decreases quality of life, diminishes multiple measures of health, and increases mortality.

A prerequisite for disease self-management in adulthood is the achievement of normal developmental milestones during adolescence, which are critical for any adolescent even without a health condition to become a functional adult. These milestones include gradual separation from parents, ability to develop dependable and fulfilling relationships with peers, developing a sense of purpose including realistic vocational goals, increasing capacity for abstract thought, and fine-tuning of executive functioning. For many adolescents with ADHD, even achieving these basic developmental milestones by their 18th birthday is a challenge, let alone having the ability to manage their ADHD independently.

Fortunately, with preparation and foresight, there is much that pediatric providers and parents can do to help adolescents with ADHD transition more effectively. It is critical to remember that transition should begin in early adolescence, *not* as the adolescent approaches his/her 18th birthday, and that efforts to help adolescents transition should be customized to their developmental stage.

IMPROVING TRANSITIONAL READINESS THROUGHOUT ADOLESCENCE: THE PROVIDER'S ROLE
Early Adolescence (Typically Age 10–12 Years)
- Teach the adolescent what ADHD is—what causes it, what its symptoms are, and how it is treated.
- During appointments start directing questions to the adolescent and not the parent. Remind the adolescent that he/she can always ask the parent for help if unsure about anything. (You may also need to remind the parent to let the adolescent try answering questions first.)

- Ensure that the adolescent has the opportunity to ask his/her own questions.
- Introduce the concept of transition and that the adolescent will eventually be responsible for 100% of their ADHD management.

Middle Adolescence (Typically Age 13–15 Years)

- Ensure that the adolescent knows the names and doses of all medications.
- The adolescent should be seen alone for at least a part of each healthcare visit.
- Adolescents should begin to share responsibility for taking their medications. Encourage the use of an alarm on their phones or another system of their devising to remember to take their medications every day. (One helpful strategy is to have the patient set an alarm on his/her cell phone during an appointment with you.) Parents should still check to ensure that medication was taken.
- A confidential psychosocial history should be periodically obtained. The "HEADS" tool (home, education, activities, drugs/diet/depression, and sex/safety) is a helpful way to perform a comprehensive psychosocial review of systems and ensure that normal adolescent developmental milestones are being achieved.
- Anticipatory guidance about the dangers of substance abuse (including the misuse and diversion of stimulant medication) and sexual risk-taking should be proactively discussed.
- Patients should be advised not to tell anyone, even good friends, that they take stimulant medication; it is better to avoid being put in a compromised position by a friend who asks to borrow medication.

Late Adolescence (Typically Age 16–17 Years)

- Most (if not all) part of the appointment should be spent with the youth alone.
- Encourage the adolescent to start booking his/her own appointments with you.
- Encourage the adolescent to start requesting his/her own medication refills.
- Encourage independent transportation (either driving or public transportation) to at least some appointments.
- Introduce the concept of a "three-sentence summary," i.e., a brief history of one's condition and comorbidities, a summary of one's current treatment plan, and current concerns or questions about one's condition and treatment.[5] For example, "I was diagnosed with

combined-type ADHD when I was 7 years and was also diagnosed with anxiety as a teenager; I was started on medication and I was on therapy throughout my adolescence, which helped. I currently take extended-release methylphenidate, 30 mg, and sertraline, 150 mg, every morning, but I have not seen a therapist since I graduated from high school. My biggest concerns are that lately I feel my ADHD medication wearing off by the early evening when I still have a lot of studying to do, and I would like to get back into therapy for my anxiety." Patients should practice stating their three-sentence summary with their pediatric care providers, which will prepare them to provide information concisely and effectively to an adult care provider in the future.
- Continue to perform a periodic comprehensive and confidential psychosocial review of systems with the adolescent, including any substance use, misuse or diversion of stimulant medication, friendships and relationships, and sexual activity.
- Engage the adolescent in discussions about the selection of an adult ADHD provider.
- Discuss upcoming insurance changes with both the adolescent and the parent, including whether the adolescent will remain on their parent's insurance or will need to apply independently for insurance.
- Encourage the adolescent to participate in joint decision-making with parents and introduce principles of consent.

Around the Time of Transition (Around 17.5–18 Years)

- Write a transition summary about the patient's ADHD history and send it in advance to the patient's new adult ADHD provider. Provide a copy to the adolescent with a reminder that he/she may need to provide this documentation to college administrators or employers in the future.
- If possible have at least one appointment with the adolescent *after* the first appointment with his/her new adult ADHD provider so that there is an opportunity to tie up any loose ends.

FINDING AN ADULT ADHD PROVIDER

It is often a challenge to find adult providers who have interest and experience in managing conditions diagnosed in childhood, such as cerebral palsy and congenital heart disease. Unfortunately, the same is true for ADHD. Most primary care for adults is completed by family physicians or internists, whose residencies do not typically include training in developmental/behavioral conditions. Furthermore, there is a paucity of primary care guidelines for the diagnosis and management of ADHD in adults.

The following strategies may assist your adolescent patients in finding an adult ADHD provider:

- Children and Adults with Attention-Deficit/Hyperactivity Disorder (CHADD), a non-profit organization, has a searchable ADHD provider directory on their website (www.chadd.org). Provider searches can be narrowed down by state, type of clinician (including family physician, psychiatrist, therapist, etc.), and age range of accepted patients.
- Adult psychiatrists may be more likely to prescribe ADHD medication than adult primary care physicians; consider transitioning your adolescent patients to both.
- If an adolescent is planning to go to college, on-campus student health clinics may offer psychiatry services including ADHD treatment. Encourage your patients to contact the student health clinics of their future colleges to determine whether these services are offered.
- Adolescent medicine physicians often see patients until their early to mid-20s. Their developmental expertise positions them well to provide comprehensive pharmacologic and nonpharmacologic ADHD treatment to transition-age youth. You can contact the Society for Adolescent Health and Medicine (www.adolescenthealth.org) to locate your nearest adolescent medicine provider.

TRANSITIONING TO ADULTHOOD, NOT JUST ADULT HEALTHCARE

Executive function is what separates adults from children, and ADHD is fundamentally a disorder of executive functioning. Many young adults with ADHD are consequently unprepared not only for managing their own healthcare but also for many other aspects of adult life, including finding a vocation, healthy relationships, financial management, and independent living. Young people with ADHD need to start practicing these critical skills in adolescence while they still have the support and protection of their families. Pediatricians should actively provide anticipatory guidance to facilitate these life skills:

- Independent living: From a relatively early age, adolescents with ADHD should be involved in household chores. By mid-adolescence, they should be expected to do their laundry, make their lunches, and clean up after themselves. They should also participate in grocery shopping and other household

errands. By late adolescence, they should be able to cook at least a few simple dishes; ideally, they should cook a meal for the whole family at least once per week.

- Financial management: Websites such as www.TheMint.org offer free online modules and games to teach children and adolescents about financial literacy. Financial literacy skills should be introduced in a developmentally appropriate manner.
  - Childhood and early adolescence
    - Allowance money should be given only if household responsibilities and chores are fulfilled.
  - Mid-adolescence
    - Adolescents should be encouraged to start a part-time job or take on odd jobs such as babysitting or mowing lawns.
    - Adolescents should open their first bank account.
  - Late adolescence
    - Adolescents should assume responsibility for making simple payments on time (e.g., paying their cell phone bills).
    - Adolescents should get their first credit card, for which they will make their own payments. They should also learn to write checks.
  - By age 18 years
    - Adolescents should make their first budget.
    - Adolescents should receive an introduction to loans, interest, mortgages, and insurance.
- Healthy relationships: By early adolescence, adolescents with ADHD should be taught about principles of sexual consent, pregnancy prevention, and STD/HIV prevention. Participation in coeducational social skills training should be encouraged; these are often offered through regional centers, community centers, or schools. The adolescent should be taught that it is healthy and normal to have friends of any gender. A part-time job, volunteer activity, or extracurricular hobby outside school can further encourage healthy and respectful peer interactions. If any romance develops, families should ensure that the relationship is positive without unhealthy elements of control or coercion and that other friendships are still maintained.
- Finding a vocation: Adolescents with ADHD should be encouraged to explore a breadth of different vocational and educational options, attend career and college fairs, and regularly speak to guidance and career counselors. They should take advantage of student internships or co-ops offered by their schools and should seek opportunities to shadow

their parents or other adults in their lives at work. It is important for adolescents with ADHD to be realistic about their strengths and weaknesses and to consider what careers would provide adequate stimulation and variety to keep them sufficiently engaged for career success and satisfaction. Careers that require hours of reading, mundane or repetitive tasks, or great attention to detail may not be the best fit, and there is nothing wrong with acknowledging this.

SUPPORTING PARENTS DURING THEIR CHILDREN'S TRANSITION

Parents are critical stakeholders in helping their adolescents to undergo transition effectively. However, sometimes it is a challenge to engage parents in transitional support because they may not trust their adolescent (especially an inattentive and impulsive adolescent) to manage independently, and it is "so much easier" to do everything themselves. It is helpful for parents to hear the rationale behind increasing transition readiness and to reassure them that transition is a gradual rather than an abrupt process spanning over the course of adolescence.

As more responsibilities in ADHD management are handed over to the adolescent suggest that parents use rewards and "natural consequences" to encourage their adolescents to follow-through until the new habits are solidified. For example, it would be reasonable for parents to allow their adolescent to borrow their car only if the adolescent has taken his/her medication, as inattentive driving is dangerous. Similarly, a parent may decide that an adolescent can only have a smartphone if he/she also uses it to maintain an up-to-date calendar tracking academic deadlines and appointments; if deadlines and appointments are missed then presumably the phone is not being used effectively and should be confiscated.

Above all, parents must resist the urge to take over if their adolescent is not following through on his/her responsibilities. Instead, they should act as sounding boards for their children to determine how to get back on track (e.g., "Looks like you haven't remembered to take your medication for the last few days—why do you think that is? Do you think that affected how you did on your math test? How could you improve your reminder system?"). Furthermore, they might need to allow their child to experience real consequences, such as losing household privileges, getting a bad grade, or paying the fee for a missed appointment themselves, so that they truly internalize the importance of adherence. It is better for young people to experience and learn the consequences of failing to manage their ADHD in adolescence than in adulthood, when they have so much more to lose.

Parents of adolescents with ADHD may find themselves "burned out" from all the transitional support they require. One potential support aid may be an ADHD coach (e.g., therapist, counselor, or other behavioral health professional) who can be hired for a monthly retainer to ensure that the adolescent is on track academically and socially. This may reduce some of the burden on the parents while allowing adolescents to have some developmentally appropriate separation from their parents.

Parents need to understand and accept the developmental trajectories of their adolescents and prepare themselves for the possibility that their children may not be ready to "leave the nest" at age 18 years. Rather than trying to launch them into adulthood on a preconceived timeline, parents should be encouraged to support what is most developmentally appropriate for their children. This may mean that they spend an extra year or two at home after high-school graduation to take a couple of community college classes, work at a part-time job, and have a little more time to develop living and self-management skills. Permitting adolescents with ADHD to have a longer transition period may increase their odds of success in adulthood.

Parents should talk to their children with ADHD about the consequences of substance abuse, sexual risk-taking, and medication misuse and diversion. Healthcare providers can give factual and medical information about these issues to adolescents, but parents can enrich these discussions by incorporating family expectations, values, cultural and spiritual beliefs, and community context.

Many young people with ADHD have a parent who also has ADHD. Sometimes, this leads to "normalization" of the consequences of ADHD within a family. Parents who have suffered the consequences of poorly controlled ADHD should be encouraged to discuss this openly with their children, including what they may wish they had done differently, and to do their best to role model good adherence to behavior modification and/or pharmacologic treatment.

WHAT TO DO IF TRANSITION IS A STRUGGLE

Despite the best efforts of parents, providers, and patients, transition to adulthood is often still a difficult period for young people with ADHD. Young adults with ADHD should be encouraged to maintain a strong support network of family and friends; online and in-person support groups are also available for youth with ADHD. Providers should monitor for comorbid anxiety and depression and ensure that these are also treated. Validation is important, and young people with ADHD need to know that they are not alone. But when they face bumps in the road as they move toward independence, providers can help them reflect on their experiences to facilitate learning, growth, and positive change.

SUMMARY

ADHD is not merely a childhood condition. Most children diagnosed with ADHD have persistent symptoms in adulthood but often abruptly lose the supports that they previously relied on to function. This can be prevented by initiating transition support in early adolescence, using rewards and natural consequences to facilitate the gradual development of self-management skills. Regular psychosocial screening and anticipatory guidance are critical to encourage normal adolescent development and reduce risk behaviors. Providers should remember that "transition" is not just about healthcare but encompasses all the responsibilities and privileges of reaching independent adulthood. Parents may need as much support as their adolescents to fulfill their roles in the transition process.

RESOURCES

CHADD provides education, advocacy, and support to parents of children with ADHD and adults with ADHD. Their website includes information about diagnosis and treatment, tip sheets for behavior modification and organizational skills, online support groups, and a directory of providers who offer ADHD-related services. Available at www.chadd.org.

Zeigler Dendy, Chris A. Teenagers with ADD and ADHD: A Guide for Parents and Professionals. Woodbine Publishing, 2006.

Ari Tuckman. More Attention, Less Deficit: Success Strategies for Adults with ADHD. Specialty Press, 2009.

Good2Go Transition Program, The Hospital for Sick Children, Toronto, ON, Canada: Provides free transition tools for adolescents and families; available at http://www.sickkids.ca/Good2Go/For-Youth-and-Families/Transition-Tools/Index.html.

Got Transition/Center for Health Care Transition Improvement: Provides free training and transition resources for professionals and families; available at www.GotTransition.org.

The Mint: A website with free online tutorials and games to teach children and adolescents financial literacy; available at www.TheMint.org.

REFERENCES

1. Sibley MH, Pelham WE, Molina BSG, et al. When diagnosing ADHD in young adults emphasize informant reports, and impairment. *J Consult Clin Psychol.* 2012;80(6):1052–1061.
2. Kessler RC, Adler L, Barkley R, et al. The prevalence and correlates of adult ADHD in the United States: results from the National Comorbidity Survey Replication. *Am J Psychiatry.* 2006;163(4):716–723.
3. Newlove-Delgado T, Ford TJ, Hamilton W, Stein K, Ukoumunne OC. Prescribing of medication for attention deficit hyperactivity disorder among young people in the Clinical Practice Research Datalink 2005-2013: analysis of time to cessation. *Eur Child Adolesc Psychiatry.* 2018;27(1):29–35.
4. Gray WN, Kavookjian J, Shapiro SK, et al. Transition to college and adherence to prescribed attention deficit hyperactivity disorder medication. *J Dev Behav Pediatr.* 2018;39(1):1–9.
5. The Hospital for Sick Children, Good2Go Program. MyHealth 3-Sentence Summary. Available from: http://www.sickkids.ca/Good2Go/For-Youth-and-Families/Transition-Tools/MyHealth-3-Sentence-Summary/Index.html.

CHAPTER 7

ADHD Accompanying Other Disorders, including Tics and Tourette Syndrome

ADHD AND ITS COEXISTENT PROBLEMS: WHAT TO TREAT FIRST

A. ADHD can be treated first in the presence of these coexistent problems:

1) oppositional defiant disorder
2) conduct disorder
3) learning problems
4) tic disorders (see subsequent section in this chapter re: ADHD, tics, and Tourette Syndrome)
5) persistent depressive disorder (dysthymia)
6) anxiety disorder, includes some milder types
   - generalized anxiety disorder
   - social anxiety
   - separation anxiety
   - school phobia (may be due to learning and attentional problems, which ADHD medications might help)

Note regarding all these problems: ADHD medications are usually given concurrently with other nonmedicinal treatments, such as cognitive behavior therapy or interpersonal therapy, anger management, parenting help, educational testing, tutoring, or other learning accommodations.

PEARL: Remember, stimulant medications can worsen anxiety.

B. ADHD plus certain other coexistent problems require treatment prioritization.

1) Significant substance abuse must be treated before adding ADHD medications.
2) Major depression with suicidal ideation must be treated first.
3) Less severe depression without suicidal ideation should be considered on a case-by-case basis.
4) Severe anxiety (e.g., panic attacks), school phobia with refusal to go, and severe separation anxiety: Probably treat anxiety first on a case-by-case basis.

PEARL: Often once the more severe concern is under treatment, e.g., depressed but no longer suicidal,

panic attacks controlled, substance abuse treated, it is then possible to cautiously add ADHD medications to the treatment program.

PEARL: ADHD medications and selective serotonin reuptake inhibitor medications are compatible for simultaneous usage.

C. Other conditions that must be treated first, prior to ADHD medication treatment:

1) psychosis
2) bipolar disorder/mania

Additional PEARL: Always first treat the condition that is most threatening or impairing.

ADHD, TICS, AND TOURETTE SYNDROME: WITH SAMUEL ZINNER, MD, FAAP
Case Vignette: ADHD With Tics

You have recently diagnosed a 9-year-old boy with ADHD, combined type. In addition to his ADHD symptoms, he has had intermittent tics, sometimes motor (eye blinking) and sometimes vocal (throat clearing).

In discussing treatment options, including behavior therapy and medications, the parents adamantly refuse a trial of stimulant medications because they read online that "Stimulant medications should not be used because they make tics worse!"

ADHD, Tics, and Tourette Syndrome: What to do!

1) Tics are movements or vocalizations that are a common problem in children and adolescents, with a prevalence (depending on whom you read) perhaps of 5%—10% in the pediatric population at any point in time. Although tics can be temporarily suppressed at times by most, though not all, patients, they are essentially involuntary and look sudden and repetitive.
   - Examples of motor tics: Eye blinking, facial grimacing, head nodding or jerking, shoulder and arm movements.

- Examples of vocal tics: Coughing, sniffing, throat clearing, grunting, chirping, and word or meaningless utterances.
2) Tic disorders are now considered to be neurodevelopmental disorders rather than neuropsychiatric disorders.
3) Tics classically start before puberty and then peak in severity at age 8–10 years, followed by a gradual decline through adolescence, although their patterns and course vary widely across people affected with tics. Sometimes they may seem to start with a symptom of some other ailment, e.g., nose sniffing due to allergic rhinitis, but then persist after the allergy improves, like a "habit" that developed. Usually, however, there is no apparent reason for the onset, and many, if not most, of the tics seem to have little relationship to physiologic or functional needs.
4) In the general pediatric population, tics tend to be simple (isolated to one muscle group (usually in the face or neck)), fairly short-lived (e.g., 1–3 months), and then disappear, often to never appear again. However, when they mimic physiologic possibilities, e.g., nose sniffing for allergy or eye blinking for visual problems, they can be a concern for parents to seek medical consultation.
5) Tics, however, can be more complicating and are therefore divided into the following types.
   - Simple motor type (involves one motor group) versus complex motor type (involves multiple motor groups, e.g., gesturing or intended action)
   - Simple vocal type (single noise, e.g., from throat) versus complex vocal type (whole statements or obscene comments)

PEARL: What is the relationship between tics and ADHD? Why is this a problem?
1) Short-lived tics are common among children (about one in every five children at some point)
2) Chronic tics (i.e., lasting a year or more) are more common in patients with ADHD than in children without ADHD, with a prevalence of 20% or so in ADHD (vs. 1% or 2% in non-ADHD).
3) The combination of ADHD and tics makes treatment (and, therefore, parental concern) more challenging, e.g., medication usage.
4) ADHD plus tics present some additional psychosocial challenges:
   - child more likely to be bullied,
   - child more prone to anxiety and/or depression,
   - child more likely to have other significant behavior concerns, such as aggression.

So what is the Tourette syndrome (TS) and what is its relationship to ADHD?

TS was named after the French neurologist Georges Gilles de la Tourette, who published nine cases of chronic tic disorder in 1885. TS is the name for a chronic tic disorder having the following characteristics:
1) Onset before age 18 years.
2) Both vocal and motor tics, not necessarily simultaneously.
3) Tics occur many times daily.
4) Persistence of tics for 12 months or longer.
Other characteristics include the following:
PEARL:
1) The majority of children with TS, perhaps half or more, have coexisting ADHD.
2) ADHD is often diagnosed prior to the tic onset.
3) The ADHD component is almost always more impairing than the tic component.
4) About 10% of patients with TS, at some point, have "coprolalia," a vocal tic symptom of derogatory or vulgar speech, swearing, etc. (despite its high publicizing, this is an unusual symptom manifestation).
5) Symptoms peak around age 10 years, then usually decline into adulthood. Although adult patients report absence of tic symptoms, videos have demonstrated that some persistence into adulthood is often present, unrecognized by others, or even the patient.
6) Another common coexisting problem can be obsessive-compulsive disorder.
7) Adolescent and adult patients with TS are usually aware of a sensory "premonition" that the tic is about to occur, sometimes described as an "urge to have the tic." This finding is helpful in the treatment called "habit reversal" (see later discussion).

PEARL: Until 25 or so years ago, it was determined (using weak data) that stimulant medication increased tic behavior and therefore such medications were contraindicated for patients with ADHD and coexistent tics, or in patients with TS and coexistent ADHD. The FDA has required a warning regarding this contraindication on all stimulant prescriptions. The Tourette Association wrote statements like "Do not let your physician prescribe stimulant medications to your T.S. child."

Although the FDA continues to issue a warning that methylphenidate (but not amphetamine) stimulants are contraindicated in people with TS, we now know, after thorough research, that the statement "Stimulant

medications cause or exacerbate tics" is essentially un-true. When one prescribes stimulant medication to a child with ADHD with coexistent tics, one of the following three things is likely to happen, which mirrors the pattern also seen in children with tics but who are not prescribed stimulants at all:
1) the tics will worsen (unlikely),
2) the tics will lessen (occasionally noted),
3) the tics will remain the same.

PEARL: When considering tic management options, first consider whether the tics are causing any problems to the child or to others. Often if the child, teacher, and peers are unconcerned, a simple approach of "watchful waiting" is appropriate. However, if any of the following scenarios occurs, treatment should be considered and probably undertaken:
1) The child is upset by the tic because of teasing, peer rejection, bullying, etc.
2) Teacher reports tic "disruptive to class," e.g., vocal outbursts.
3) Physical issues, such as picking at skin, bleeding, infection.
4) School avoidance due to tic.

Children with ADHD and tics, or TS with coexistent ADHD, should all receive the same thorough diagnostic evaluation for ADHD described in chapter 3. Special emphasis should be made on looking for causes of distress in the child (e.g., school, peer relations), which clearly can intensify tic symptoms. For example, a subtle learning problem, previously unnoted, may, with remedial help, result in lessening of the tic symptoms. Rectifying an unhealthy peer relationship or family dysfunction might have the same positive effect.

Treatment for ADHD with tics, or TS with ADHD, should follow the same multimodal treatment for ADHD already discussed in chapter 4.
1) Education regarding ADHD: In kids with tics, a thorough discussion regarding the natural course of the tic disorder is an important factor.
2) School accommodations: A subtle learning problem possibly needs to be identified and remediated. Also, Individuals with Disabilities Education Act and Section 504 laws can be utilized to provide appropriate educational accommodations.
3) Behavior therapy
   - Along with behavior modifications for the ADHD, in the children with ADHD, tics, or TS, it is extremely important to screen for anxiety, depression, and obsessive-compulsive disorder and treat appropriately (such as with cognitive behavior therapy and/or medication).
   - For TS consider "habit reversal therapy," which uses the child's premonitory urge to have the tic either to perform a movement or sound that is likely to be unrecognized as a tic or to progressively learn strategies of increasingly tolerable tic suppression while also reducing or avoiding situations that trigger or exacerbate tic behavior. For example, to replace the shoulder jerking with an ear scratching, which would not be noted as a tic.
4) Helpful organizations for the parents and child (books, meetings, etc.):
   - CHADD (Children and Adults with Attention-Deficit/Hyperactivity Disorder),
   - TAA (Tourette Association of America).
5) Medications (several general principles are listed here; see section on Case Scenarios in chapter 4. [what to do when your favorite ADHD medication doesn't work.])
   - When targeting ADHD symptoms for medication treatment use stimulants first, following guidelines in the ADHD chapter. If not successful with the first stimulant then repeat the trial with another type of stimulant.
   - If tics worsen on both types of stimulant medication, particularly if this is dose-related, consider a smaller dose of stimulant and add an α-agonist (e.g., clonidine or guanfacine, or the long-acting forms Kapvay and Intuniv). This might give better ADHD control as well as lessen tics.
   - Or one could stop the stimulant medication and just try a long-acting α-agonist.
   - Or one could stop the stimulant and try atomoxetine.
   - Remember that both α-agonists and atomoxetine are second-level ADHD medications and are less likely to bring optimal control of ADHD symptoms when used alone compared with the stimulants.
   - Adding smaller than therapeutic doses of stimulants to the atomoxetine or α-agonists often works well.
   - Atypical antipsychotic medication, although helpful for controlling tic symptoms, should not be used except in extremely complex cases because of the adverse side effects of these medications when compared with the relative risk of the tics.

See chapter on Scenarios.

CHAPTER 8

Enhancing Resilience in a Child With ADHD

MICHAEL JELLINEK, MD, FAACAP

Resilience is defined as the capability of a strained body to recover its size and shape after deformation caused by stress. How a specific material "bounces back" depends both upon its composition and the nature, duration, frequency, intensity, and temperature of the deforming force (e.g., the tragic "O-ring" failure of the Challenger disaster). Similarly, the factors that contribute to a child's development, such as genetics, personality, and parenting, will influence how that child reacts to stresses. In a child with ADHD, resilience is the psychological process of adapting well or "bouncing back" in the face of adversity or significant stress. As ADHD is a 24-h condition a child with ADHD faces varying levels of stress almost every waking hour (as well as potential sleep disturbance). A child with ADHD will face many more and often more serious stressors than most children and is more likely to be vulnerable to stresses that might otherwise not require resilience.

Inattention may impact listening to a parent trying to get the household up and running in the morning. If the child is simply inattentive, he/she may miss a request or instruction, get distracted and not brush his/her teeth, or not bring all that is needed for a day at school. If the child has additional organizational difficulties, he/she may not be consistent in getting dressed or other age-appropriate tasks. If physically hyperactive, the child may be running around the house, bothering siblings, and creating a sense of chaos. Each aspect of the child's problem calls forth more suggestions, more criticisms, more exasperation, and likely more tension. Each correction is a "compressive stress," a feeling of adversity or even inadequacy that requires a "bounce back" to face the next few minutes.

Imagine a school day for a child with ADHD. Would a teacher making four "pay attention" comments in an hour be excessive or unusual? In a 6-h day that would be 24 corrections. Add after-school activities or sports team for 2 h, and we are up to 32. At home, maybe four before school and four between dinner and bedtime, which is likely a conservative assumption. A typical first grader would then experience 7200 comments in a 180-day school year, plus whatever number, probably lower, in the remaining 185 days. In my experience, 10,000 comments every year is more likely an underestimate than an exaggeration.

Those trying to help the child with ADHD, having every good intention, are highly valued influential people in the child's life—parents, siblings, teachers, after-school counselors, and coaches. The people who are pleading, repeatedly asking, or criticizing the child are those that give interpersonal meaning to a child's life and serve as umpires as the child develops an identity and self-esteem.

So we have defined the issue. A child with ADHD will likely hear 10,000 comments/corrections from meaningful, well-intentioned, and highly valued adults every year. Supporting a material that can bounce back from 10,000 compressions or stresses a year requires a serious, thoughtful, and sustained effort.

What are the factors we have to take into account? How severe are the compressions or stresses? How clear are they, not just in wording, but in the child's understanding? How much does the child experience these comments as a negative judgment about them as a person? How much anger is built into the wording and tone of these comments? What is the overall balance in their life between blame, sense of failure and criticism versus praise, areas of strength, and a sense of success? How many areas of their life are involved? Inattention? Physical hyperactivity? Organizational difficulties? Learning disabilities? How severe are each of these different factors?

What are some of the core characteristics of the child burdened by ADHD and one or more difficulties? Is their temperament from birth optimistic or pessimistic? Are they flexible adapting to new situations or rigid? Is any learning problem subtle and a lower priority or a critical deficiency that the whole class sees every day? Do they have built-in compensating skills such as being socially adept, having an acknowledged area of strength, or higher intelligence?

Beyond the built-in genetic and temperamental "bounce-back" abilities that a child may or may not have from birth, what can a parent or teacher do to enhance resiliency?

1. **Empathy supports resilience.** Does the child feel that someone important in his/her lives, a parent, teacher, or counselor, understands the stress he/she experiences every day and appreciates how hard he/she is trying to meet expectations. Given the genetic patterns of ADHD, one-third to a half of all children will have a close relative, often a father, who had or has ADHD. A father sharing his struggle and memories with his child with ADHD is very meaningful, and appreciating his child's efforts supports the ability to "bounce back" and self-esteem. Empathy builds a warm supportive relationship with an adult, which is a critical protective factor and makes a child feel "connected" and valued. An empathic relationship with an adult, hopefully a parent, merits the highest priority on this list.

2. **Customize expectations for the child.** The formula for setting reasonable expectations is to take the child's genetic strengths and weaknesses, add ADHD, include any added factors such as learning disabilities or any other family stressors (poverty, parental tensions, chronic disease, etc.), then subtract 10% from their peak abilities, and the result equals a reasonable expectation. Why subtract 10%? Two reasons. First, none of us "do our best" all the time and expecting us to "always do your best" is not possible or reasonable. Instead a "do your best" orientation evokes lower self-esteem and interpersonal distance. Second, it is safer to underestimate a bit and encourage a greater feeling of success than overestimate and attribute a sense of failure to a very good if not maximal effort. Remember, we are talking about a child facing 10,000 compressions or stressors a year.

3. **Medications play a role in resilience.** Stimulants decrease ADHD symptoms and in turn dramatically lower the number of criticisms experienced by the child every day. Key adults, parents, teachers, and coaches will change the ratio of criticisms to praise, with the children feeling better about themselves, which in turn may enhance the relationship with the adult and strengthen the ability to "bounce back." If medication results in fewer and more controllable symptoms, the resulting enhancement of resilience is a substantial benefit.

4. **Building on a child's strengths, such as sports, music, and computer skills, enhances resilience.** As we wish the child to be whole, as good as they can be, we naturally focus on remediating weaknesses and sometimes try to remedy multiple weaknesses at the same time or in rapid sequence. Remediation for the child means dwelling on or highlighting areas of weakness and may get an extra jolt of emotional energy from every parent's wish to have a normal, high-functioning child. Of course, we should try to remedy areas of weakness, but we need to recognize that remediation is experienced as another compression or stress that requires bouncing back. None of us would like to attend 2 or 3 h of remediation every day. Most of us like to practice what we do well, what others admire and praise, and to remember our strength when "compressed." Children with ADHD need to feel good about some area, actually very good, to bounce back from weaknesses. In adult life, once we reach a minimal standard, few of us choose to work in areas that highlight our deficiencies; instead, we choose and enjoy areas that engage our strengths.

5. **Human and technical support can help.** A tutor experienced in ADHD and learning problems can support a child with ADHD. Beyond the technical assistance with homework, test preparation, and organization, many tutors develop a very positive relationship with the child. A tutor adds an empathic adult who values the child, which will contribute to resiliency. Furthermore, some children with ADHD benefit from the capabilities of a smartphone with scheduling, reminders, and other applications as well as by using a computer in the classroom, which may be enormously helpful to certain children.

6. Children with ADHD are often exhausted by the all-day effort to perform well in school and repeatedly bouncing back from adversity is draining. **Giving a child with ADHD "downtime" or restorative activities after school and on weekends supports resiliency.** For example, allowing them to play videogames, enjoy an after-school sport, participate in an art class, watch TV—anything that is easy, pleasurable—will support resiliency. Every child and especially those with ADHD need periods of "senseless fun" where there are not right answers and no implicit or explicit achievable goal.

7. **A well-planned summer program with remediation kept to a minimum also supports resiliency.** Looking forward to a family vacation, summer camp, especially a sleepaway camp that fits the

child's interests and personality, is a refuge. Helping a child build skills and friendships, having some senseless fun, and further reinforcing a positive relationship with parents or counselors is a good preparation for another demanding school year.

8. **A meaningful framework helps a child with ADHD.** School is one of the most difficult settings for children, as it tests weaknesses and vulnerabilities in different academic and social areas for many hours each day. Parents should point out what is interesting in school, what progress is being made, and where school efforts may lead in terms of personal interests or interests. In the long term, many children with ADHD will then be much happier out of school over the summer and when they join the working world. If they are guided to pick areas where they have strengths, feel successful, and fit their capacities, then they feel a sense of relief and become a valued hard worker when unburdened by the "compressive forces" of school.

9. **A child with ADHD should have an annual review** that should not only consider academic progress but also look at peer relationships, self-esteem, and positive activities and should evaluate the compression/praise ratio in the context of the child's resiliency.

Over the course of childhood and adolescence in a child with ADHD, resiliency, the ability to bounce back from compression, stress, or adversity, is the source of energy for trying again, for grit, and for persistence. **Parents and other adults can support resilience by setting empathic reasonable expectations, having a caring relationship that communicates how much the child is valued, and supporting the child being connected to people and to areas of strength.** Children with ADHD will get knocked down much more often than other children and supporting resiliency will help them get up after every stress.

CHAPTER 9

Anxiety Disorders Secondary or Coexistent With ADHD

THE MENTAL HEALTH INTERVIEW

Those of us trained in medicine learned a diagnostic approach starting with the identification of what is called the "chief complaint." This was the presenting symptom, be it headache, stomach ache, fatigue, whatever. Then we learned to ask many questions about the how, when, where etc. of that complaint.

Taking a mental health history follows that same outline. We identify, if possible, what is the chief concern for the appointment and then ask the how, when, and where types of questions, obviously directing those questions more toward psychosocial concerns than to physical symptoms. In our educational programs at The Resource for Advancing Children's Health (REACH) Institute, e.g., the Patient-Centered Mental Health in Pediatric Primary Care course, we use a lot of mnemonics to simplify the process, e.g., COLDER is used to describe the components of the mental health interview.

C: What are the **Characteristics** of the concern? Sadness? Fear/panic? Anger?

O: **Onset**. When does the problem occur? For example, what am I doing usually when I have this concern?

L: **Location.** Where does the problem (anxiety, fear, etc.) occur? School? Home? Work? During soccer games, tests, etc. When I'm alone? In a group?

D: **Duration.** How long does it last? A few minutes, hours, days?

E: **Exacerbation**. What makes it worse? Is it impairing? i.e., keeps me from functioning as I want to or should do.

R: **Relief.** What makes it better? Must I leave or avoid the situation? What can I do to make it better?

The Mental Health Card can be used as a prompt right at your desk to guide you through the interview process.

Along with the abovementioned, always remember to get a full history of all the other aspects of the child's life, not only the growth and development, review of systems, hospitalizations, serious illness, etc. but also the complete information about the psychosocial areas that might be crucial to understand the mental health concern, things including school achievement, family and peer relationships, family history (separation, divorce, etc.), family history of mental issues such as anxiety/depression, bipolar disorder, self-esteem, previous counseling or testing, etc. Also obtain information on the child's interests, skills, hobbies, goals, etc. Any concerns about substance abuse, suicidal ideation? REMEMBER TO ASK ABOUT THE CHILD'S STRENGTHS, WHICH WE CAN BUILD UPON.

See Chapter 1 for a helpful Parent questionnaire we developed for patients with academic and behavioral concerns, which will elicit much of this information prior to the first appointment. Although copyrighted feel free to use it to fit your needs, as long as credit is given to us, the developers The Mental Health Card (see below image) is a guide to the mental health interview.

Mental Health Card

SOAP

For children under 11 y/o, meet with parent and child together to discuss chief concern.
Then meet alone with child for at least five minutes.
For adolescents, consider meeting with adolescent first.

CHIEF CONCERN
If not specific, consider starting with school and social history

SYMPTOM-SPECIFIC HISTORY
DESCRIPTION: (what it is...get concrete examples, including)
Time Frame: Initial event? Persistent/intermittent? Duration? Cyclical? Prolonged hiatus?
When: Global? Triggered? Persistent/intermittent? Cyclical? Prolonged hiatus?
Setting: School? Home? Alone? With others? Who?
Intensity?
What makes it better? What makes it worse?
RESPONSE:
How do you deal with it?
Is there anything that YOU do that makes it better?
Adaptive skills?
EtOH? Self-medicating?
Is there anything that YOU do that makes it worse?
IMPAIRMENT:
Tell me how bad it gets/got...describe it to me (time, place, situation)
What's the worst it ever got?
Depression?
Suicidal thoughts?
Aggression?
What does it stop you from doing?

COLDER
Characteristics
Onset
Location
Duration
Exacerbation
Relief

REVIEW OF SYSTEMS (e.g., Mood, Sleep, Appetite, Energy, Concentration, Anxiety, Aggression, etc)

BIRTH, DEVELOPMENTAL AND BEHAVIORAL HISTORY

RELEVANT MEDICAL HISTORY (include meds/otc)

SCHOOL HISTORY
Academics? Behavior? Extra services? Recent changes?
May need to get parental permission to communicate with school

SOCIAL HISTORY
Living environment
Trauma History, including witnessed domestic violence
Friends (changes, new, withdrawal)
Substance use
Functioning, strengths, interests

TARGETED FAMILY HISTORY

SAFETY--danger to self, danger to others
Is the home safe (no guns, access to Tylenol, etc)?
Safety Plan/Contract: (What is the plan if thoughts of harming self or others emerge?)

LAB VALUES/TOOLS

ASSESSMENT/DIAGNOSIS

TREATMENT OPTIONS (consider guidelines or algorithm)

(Reprinted with permission from The Resource for Advancing Children's Health (REACH) Institute, Patient-Centered Mental Health in Pediatric Primary Care (PPP) program copyright.)

ANXIETY DISORDERS
Case Vignette: Anxiety

Elena is a 14-year-old girl brought in to the clinic by her mother because of recent symptoms of headache, insomnia, and fatigue. Mom wonders if she might have "mono" (which she herself had as a teenager).

Elena was diagnosed with ADHD, inattentive type, 2 years prior, when she entered middle school. Problems then included not only inattentiveness but also failure to complete her homework on time. She was given ADHD medication and attends a study skills class. A 504 plan was arranged that provides up-front seating, taking tests in the library where she is not as distracted, and 24-h grace period to turn in her homework, in case she forgets it at home. All of this has been very helpful, and she is now described as a "good student." Recently, however, she has again struggled getting her work done on time, and she is "very worried" that her grades are suffering.

Mom says she has always been a shy child. For example, she is hesitant to try new things, sometimes even appearing anxious, and this concern has increased in the recent months.

Mom says she herself recalls many of these same issues during her adolescent years, and even recalls having some "panic attacks."

Anxiety Disorders in Children and Adolescents

Anxiety disorders in children and adolescents are not rare. In fact, they are quite common. Research suggests an overall incidence of 8%–10%, but in select high-risk groups, such as ADHD, the risk may go as high as 20%–25%.

First remember the normal developmental stages often accompanied by anxiety:

Nine months: Parent leaving, hands infant to a strange adult, infant cries.

Preschool: Separation from home (may even lead to aggressive behavior).

Childhood: Test anxiety, performing before others (often called "shyness").

Adolescence: Need for peer identification (look like others—clothes, hair, etc.).

Young adult: Leaving home, college, new job, transition to independence.

All these symptom stages, although common and part of "normal" development, can be exaggerated, or prolonged, at which point they may become an impairment.

What are the symptoms of anxiety?

1) Physical complaints: Headache, stomach ache, etc.

2) Behavioral and/or emotional reactions presenting as
   - school refusal
   - decreased attention span
   - sleep disorders
   - fear of specific social situations, e.g., crowds, performance, etc.
   - obsessions/compulsions

3) In summary, a reluctance in what would be considered the normal events of growing up.

The differential diagnosis includes anxiety-producing conditions that involve both physical/medical conditions and emotional/behavioral disorders.

Medical	Emotional/Behavioral
Hyperthyroidism	• ADHD
	• Autistic spectrum disorder
	• General anxiety disorder
Cardiac disorders	
Asthma	Bipolar disorder
Diabetes	Learning problems
Seizures	Depression
Pediatric autoimmune neuropsychiatric disorders associated with *Streptococcus* (PANDAS) syndrome and pediatric acute-onset neuropsychiatric syndrome (PANS)	Bullying
Migraine	Pregnancy
Drug abuse (street drugs)	Obsessive-compulsive disorder
Caffeine abuse	Posttraumatic stress disorder
	Adjustment reactions
Anxiety can occur commonly as a genetic family disorder	Other threatening causes

How does one proceed to assess for anxiety in a child or adolescent?

1) Take a thorough medical, behavioral, developmental history.
   - Many of the abovementioned conditions will be ruled out by the history.
   - Ask the parent (and older child/adolescent), "Tell me what you mean when you talk about anxiety."
   - Clarify and delineate the nature of the anxiety: When, where, and how it presents; what precipitates it; what makes it better or worse; what symptoms it produces; duration; severity.

PEARL: NOTE THE DEGREE TO WHICH IT CAUSES FUNCTIONAL IMPAIRMENT!

2) Perform a physical examination, including height, weight, blood pressure, pulse, etc.

3) Use a rating scale to quantitatively measure the degree of anxiety.

Note: The Screen for Child Anxiety Disorders rating scale can be scored to measure the degree of anxiety (total) or subscored to measure the "type" of anxiety, e.g., separation anxiety, social anxiety, school anxiety, panic disorder.

PEARL: Because these subtypes overlap and the treatment is not necessarily specific for each subtype, the scoring by subtype is not always helpful or indicated.

PEARL: In an adolescent with significant anxiety consider using the CRAFFT screening tool for substance abuse, which can be a frequent and significant cause for the anxiety.

Treatment of Anxiety Disorders

If the anxiety is significant (i.e., functionally impairing to some major aspect of life such as school performance, social or family or job interactions, or any other major activity) treatment should be considered.

There are two evidence-based treatments for anxiety in children and adolescents:

1) cognitive behavior therapy (CBT),
2) specific medications.

The definitive research study in this population is the Child/Adolescent Anxiety Multimodal Study (CAMS), an NIH study of 488 youth, aged 7–17 years, with anxiety (excluding OCD) over a 12-week period and randomized to one of the four treatment groups:

1) CBT
2) Medication (sertraline, SER)
3) Combination of CBT and SER (Comb)
4) Placebo (PBO)

Using the Clinical Global Inventory response rate to measure efficacy of each treatment group, reduction of anxiety occurred at different rates:

Comb (81%) > CBT (60%) = SER (55%) > PBO (24%)

Results obtained using the Pediatric Anxiety Rating Scale were

Comb > SER = CBT > PBO

Medication and CBT were about equally effective, but the combination of the two was somewhat more effective.

Treatment pearls

- Mild cases: Education about anxiety focused on parent and child/adolescent, and monitor and if symptoms persist start with CBT.
- Moderate to severe cases: Consider combined therapy.
- Partial response to CBT: Add medication.
- Unavailability of CBT (due to cost or lack of trained therapists): Use medication.
- Follow progress of functional impairment, not just symptom reduction.
- Titration of medications: "Start low, go slow!"
- Medication treatment should be continued at least for 6 months, or longer as indicated.

Description of cognitive behavior therapy. PEARL: CBT (compared to interpersonal psychotherapy) has the strongest evidence base from randomized controlled trials in school-aged children and youth with anxiety and depression.

CBT is a specific treatment protocol in which therapists are trained and certified in CBT (some therapists say they do CBT but are not trained or certified).

CBT involves several well-delineated steps (and may take several months):

1) Education about the disorder, treatment, prognosis, etc.
2) Training in symptom management, e.g., relaxation techniques.
3) Cognitive restructuring, mostly eliminating negative thoughts and anticipations, e.g., a noise on the roof is more likely a bird or squirrel, not a burglar.
4) Desensitization by gradual exposure techniques, e.g., fear of driving on freeway is initiated in very small steps, not during rush hour.
5) Relapse prevention planning.

Medications

1) FDA-approved medications for use in children and adolescents for the treatment of generalized anxiety disorder

Selective Serotonin Reuptake Inhibitors	Starting Dosage (Daily in mg)
Fluoxetine (Prozac), ≥7 y/o	5–10
Fluvoxamine (Luvox), ≥7 y/o	25
Sertraline (Zoloft), ≥6 y/o	12.5–25 (used in CAMS)
Serotonin-Norepinephrine Reuptake Inhibitors	
Duloxetine (Cymbalta), ≥7 y/o	30mg (age 7–17)

2) Benzodiazepines
- No evidence (controlled studies) is useful in childhood anxiety disorders (although beneficial in adults).
- Used sometimes as adjunct short-term treatment in conjunction with selective serotonin reuptake inhibitors (SSRIs) in severe anxiety to facilitate CBT.
- Contraindicated in adolescents with substance abuse (may become addictive).

PEARL: Anxiety occurs commonly in ADHD (20%–25%). It is often secondary to the poor school performance associated with ADHD. When the child's school performance improves, with appropriate treatment of ADHD, along with school interventions, the anxiety may improve and not require any medication treatment.

On the other hand, anxiety can occasionally be worsened by stimulant medication.

SEE CHAPTER 8 ON TREATMENT OF DEPRESSION RE: SSRI DOSAGES, TITRATION, TAPERING, SIDE-EFFECTS, ETC.

SSRI medications and ADHD stimulant medications can be used together, if necessary.
- Monitor both ADHD and anxiety when treating both the disorders simultaneously.
- The abovementioned is adapted from PPP course workbook, The REACH Institute, and faculty lecture notes.

Reference: Connolly SD, Bernstein GA. Work group on quality issues. Practice parameter for the assessment and treatment of children and adolescents with anxiety disorders. *J Am Acad Child Adolesc Psychiatry* 2007;46(2):267–283.

IS IT ADOLESCENT SOCIAL ANXIETY DISORDER OR SHYNESS?

Case Vignette: Jason is a 16-year-old adolescent who was diagnosed at age 12 years with ADHD, inattentive type. Symptoms then were mostly inattentiveness and failure to complete assignments and projects in a timely manner. He subsequently improved remarkably on ADHD medication, study skills classes, and a homework tutor.

Mom raises a current concern, namely, his "excessive shyness." He has not yet attended a school dance, despite being urged by friends. He dropped out of speech class when peers laughed (he thought inappropriately) at his first speech.

"He has always been very shy," his mother notes, e.g., when he was sent to the blackboard to show his work, even though he is an excellent math student. She shares that she identifies with him because she had the same issues as a teenager.

Many children and especially adolescents, when called upon to interact in various social situations, will either be reluctant or actually refuse. The parent or the other adult involved might respond with, "Oh, he (she) is just shy," and certainly "shyness" might be an almost endearing personality trait. When does "shyness" really raise the question of a possibly impairing social anxiety disorder?

We have already in the beginning of this current chapter 9 on Anxiety, described the anxiety of certain developmental stages, e.g., nine months fear of strangers, preschool fear of separation from parents, etc. In this chapter, we are discussing the period of adolescence where many environmental factors converge on the adolescent as anxiety producers, such as school, body change, and peer relations. When is the term "shyness" no longer appropriate?

A) Definition: Social anxiety Disorder is a condition in which a person becomes very anxious, or even panicky, when exposed to the observation of others and perceives he or she is being rejected or looked at negatively.

Some other characteristics:
1) The fear reaction is disproportionate to the situation causing it.
2) It happens repeatedly when the provoking situation reoccurs.
3) The symptoms can be painful as well as impairing to the individual's functioning (e.g., social behavior).
4) The symptoms are not due to another medical or mental condition.
5) The symptoms result in future avoidance behaviors of the provoking situation.

B) Incidence and demographics
1) The overall incidence of social anxiety disorder is about 7% (both adults and adolescents, but studies show it varies from 7% to 19%).
2) It is more common in females than males, ~2:1.
3) It is more common in older adolescents than in younger adolescents.
4) The more intense the social fears, or the number of different fears, the more likely the clinical course will be more severe and the more likely

there will be more significant impairment and/ or psychiatric comorbidity.

5) **PEARL:** The impairment of social anxiety disorder can profoundly impact school achievement, e.g., finishing high school or attending college.

6) The median age of onset of symptoms is around 13 years.

C) Social anxiety disorder vs. shyness (see below table)

1) Both share the same fear, or discomfort, of certain social situations.

2)Each can evoke similar bodily responses, e.g., lack of eye contact, limitation of speech.

3) **PEARL:** Social anxiety disorder affects fewer individuals than shyness but is associated with greater impairment and possible psychiatric comorbidity.

4) Some persons having social anxiety disorder are not considered "shy" by peers.

5) Core distinctions between shyness and social anxiety disorder are listed in the following table (remember, exceptions occur!).

	Shyness	Social Anxiety Disorder
Conceptualization	Normative temperament	Psychiatric disorder
Prevalence	Fairly common, ~50% of youth	Less common, ~9% of youth
Impairment	None to minimal	Significant
Associated Psychiatric Disorders	• Marginal risk for anxiety disorder • Even less for other psychiatric disorders	Greater risk for mood, anxiety, behavior, and substance abuse disorders

Used permission from M. Burstein.

D) Key questions the clinician can ask to help differentiate shyness from social anxiety disorder (per M. Burstein):

1) Does the adolescent feel marked distress because of fear or anxiety of social situations?

2) Does the adolescent's fear or anxiety of social situations significantly interfere with his/her ability to form and maintain relationships with peers, succeed academically, or have meaningful family relationships?

3) Does the fear or anxiety in the face of social situations persist, even after some experience with these situations?

PEARL: Positive responses to any of these questions would suggest the need for further assessment of social anxiety disorder.

E) Treatment

1) Counseling, e.g., CBT, social effectiveness training for children with social phobia, the Coping Cat.

2) SSRI medication.

F) Recommendation

Please refer to the earlier section in this chapter 9 re: screening, diagnosis, and treatment of anxiety.

Resource: M. Burstein, et al. Social phobia and subtypes in the national comorbidity survey-adolescent supplement; prevalence, correlates, and comorbidity. *JAACAP* September 2011.

CHAPTER 10

Obsessive-Compulsive Disorder

CASE VIGNETTE

Anne is a 14-year-old adolescent female who is brought in by her mom for her quarterly ADHD check-back appointment. She was diagnosed with ADHD, inattentive type, 2 years prior by her pediatrician, when school reported that she "daydreamed" a lot in class and "chatted incessantly" with her neighbors instead of doing her classwork. After assessment and diagnosis, she was begun on Concerta, titrated up to 36 mg/d, with good response. Teachers were very pleased, mom said. It was like "night and day."

At today's appointment, however, mom reports that a previous concern, milder initially, is now worsening. She has always been a "perfectionist," mom says, much unlike her older brother who also has ADHD and whom Anne describes as a "slob." Mom says her perfectionism is "getting out of hand," e.g., she awakens each day at 4:30 a.m. because it takes her 2 h to get her hair "just right." Teachers have stated she occasionally seems sleepy in class. Her homework "takes forever" because if she makes the slightest mistake she tears it up and starts over. She locks her bedroom and refuses to let her younger siblings in, because they "mess it up."

Recently she has "almost developed a fetish about cleanliness," mom says, taking a shower both before and after school, washing her hands after touching any object in the home, and refusing to eat out with the family due to fear of "catching a germ."

Obsessive-compulsive disorder (OCD) is best defined as a chronic disorder characterized by a person having recurrent thoughts (worries, concerns, etc.) that are manifested as obsessions, which are relieved, or lessened, only if the person responds with certain behaviors (compulsions). The response relieves the immediate stress of the obsession, but unfortunately the relief it produces is short-lived, thus requiring repetitive responses, e.g., anxiety that the door is unlocked causes repetitive rechecking of the lock, possibly 25 or more times a day, to relieve the stress of an unlocked door. It is estimated that a person with OCD will spend an hour or more daily on such a repetitive behavior response. Obviously, such obsessive-compulsive behavior can result in significant problems or impairment in the person's performance of daily life.

A partial list of obsessional type behaviors includes the following.

1) Fixation on one's own body: Shape, appearance, cleanliness, neatness, flaws, etc.
2) Picking at the skin, hairpulling, chewing finger nails.
3) Accumulating possessions, often of little or no value, excessively (hoarding).
4) Repetitive behaviors, such as checking the door lock.
5) Not being able to "forgive and forget," e.g., other's mistakes, or "being wronged" by others, holding grudges.
6) Fear of being contaminated by germs, possible diseases.
7) Being worrisome, always thinking of the worst possible outcomes, even unrealistically.
8) Need for everything (including objects, events, etc.) to be sequential, orderly, symmetrical, etc. Not left to haphazard or chance.
9) Always desirous of being in control, leaving nothing to chance.
10) Fixation on certain attitudes or beliefs.

Obsessive-compulsive traits can be seen in other mental health conditions, e.g., anxiety, depression, ADHD, autism, Tourette syndrome, as a coexistent disorder.

OCDs can be distinguished from normal type behaviors or preoccupations by their excessiveness and persistence over time; for example, washing hands before eating can be considered a "normal" ritual, but handwashing 25–50 times daily is obviously both excessive and impairing.

Obsessive symptoms can be divided into several separate categories:

1) Fear of germs and/or contamination: Results in excessive handwashing or cleanliness.
2) Need for symmetry: Arranging and rearranging, counting and recounting, reordering, etc. Need for exactness in grouping and sequencing.

3) Tendency to overanalyze: One's thoughts, behaviors, relationships, events.
4) Unwarranted fears: Excessive worrying about harm to oneself or others, worrying about potentially harmful events, need for constant and/or repetitive reassurances.
5) Need for self-control: Having strict self-rules, taboos, unacceptable thoughts, behaviors, e.g., sexual or religious.
6) History of tic disorders (motor or vocal): About 30% of patients with OCD have life-long tic disorders.

In summary, the pathogenesis of an OCD can be viewed as recurrent thoughts or urges that are both undesired and unacceptable, cause distress, and make the person try to either ignore or suppress the stressful stimulus by performing a stress-relieving response. Unfortunately, the relief is temporary and requires repetitive efforts to relieve the stressful stimulus. As with all mental health conditions, other diagnostic traits must be met:

1) The signs and symptom traits have to be impairing to at least one major life activity: Peers, family, home, school, vocation, etc.
2) The impairment symptom should consume at least 1 h per day.
3) The symptoms should be caused neither by other medical conditions nor by an adverse side effect of a medication.

Other diagnostic features include the following:

1) Many patients with OCD have dysfunctional beliefs, e.g., inflated self-worth or perfectionism.
2) Frequently, patients with OCD have a poor insight regarding possible outcomes if certain activities or rituals are not repetitively performed.
3) Frequency of OCD behaviors can be defined:
   Mild, occupies about 1 h per day.
   Moderate, occupies 1–3 h per day.
   Severe, almost the entire day is occupied by intrusions requiring compulsive responses.

There are also associated features in patients with OCD:

1) Many patients exhibit more than one symptom trait.
2) Symptoms come and go. Patients may avoid situations that cause distress.
3) Patients may use alcohol or drugs to lessen symptoms.
4) There is a wide variation in how individuals respond. For example, one person might feel uneasy, whereas another might have a panic attack or one person might have just a feeling of distrust, whereas another person might manifest total avoidance behavior.

Epidemiology of OCD:

1) Incidence in the United States is 1%–2%.
2) Lifetime prevalence in children and adolescents is 2%–4% (~1% at any given moment, Pediatric OCD Treatment Study).
3) Mean age at onset: Late adolescence (may occur earlier but not noted by parents or other adults, and children may be unable to articulate their feelings).
4) Tendency for chronic course if starting in childhood, with continuation through adult life.
5) Rare onset after the age of 35–40 years or so.
6) Symptoms more variable in children and adolescents, and more "fixed" in adults.
7) Males are more prone to earlier symptoms of OCD and more likely to have related secondary symptoms, e.g., tics.
8) Children often manifest symptoms related to fears of death and dying.
9) OCD occurs in all cultural/ethnic groups around the world.

There are several risk factors for the development of OCD:

1) Strongly genetic: Twice more common in adult first-degree relatives, and even higher in childhood-onset cases.
2) Traumatic events, physical, sexual, etc. can trigger OCD symptoms and traits.
3) One unique form, pediatric autoimmune neuropsychiatric disorders associated with *Streptococcus* (PANDAS) syndrome, is presumed to be a delayed reaction to streptococcal infection, according to some investigators, but this belief is controversial and not definitively proven.

PROGNOSIS IN PATIENTS DIAGNOSED WITH OBSESSIVE-COMPULSIVE DISORDER

Patients with OCD can have significant impairment in areas of life function due to the excessive amount of time and energy used by the obsession and the resultant compulsion. By definition, one needs at least 1 h consumed by the obsession/compulsion to qualify for the diagnosis of OCD. "Moderately severe" cases consume 1–3 h per day, and "severe" cases consume almost an entire day for the intrusions (obsessions) and the responses to them (compulsions). So the impact on quality and quantity of meaningful life can be impacted greatly.

The impact on the family, siblings, parents, and children can also be enormous, just because of the time factors. The fallout on school achievement and job performance can also be very pronounced. At times, it is so pronounced that the adolescent severely impacted cannot reach functional adulthood. Suicidality increases markedly, felt by about 50% of patients with OCD, and one-half of those make a suicidal gesture.

DIAGNOSIS OF OBSESSIVE-COMPULSIVE DISORDER

The following are included in the diagnosis of OCD:

Thorough medical history, including presenting symptom, review of systems, past medical/developmental/educational/behavioral/family histories (presumably from both patient and parents).

Mental health interview (see Chapter 9) utilizing the Mental Health Card.

Physical examination, to rule out other health problems and observe for evidence of nail biting, hairpulling, excoriation, tic behaviors, etc.

Screening tools: e.g., Screen for Child Anxiety Disorders for anxiety disorders, Patient Health Questionnaire 9 for depression, CRAFFT for substance abuse, Yale-Brown Obsessive-Compulsive Scale (Y-BOCS).

Laboratory tests: As indicated, e.g., CBC, Chem. panel, thyroid, drug screen.

Imaging: Not clinically specific or helpful at this time.

DIFFERENTIAL DIAGNOSIS OF OBSESSIVE-COMPULSIVE DISORDER

Differential diagnosis of OCD includes several diagnoses with overlapping symptom traits: e.g., anxiety, depression, tic disorders, ADHD, Tourette syndrome, PANDAS syndrome/pediatric acute-onset neuropsychiatric syndrome, bipolar disorder, even psychoses, substance abuse, eating disorders. These diagnoses can be not only overlapping but also coexistent with the OCD diagnosis. All of this requires thorough diagnostic efforts.

TREATMENT (EVIDENCE BASED)

1) Psychotherapy

   Cognitive behavior therapy (CBT): Special type called "exposure and response prevention"

   Therapy for tics: Habit reversal therapy and/or medications
   (see chapter 7 on ADHD, tics, and Tourette Syndrome)

2) Medications (FDA approved)

   Tricyclic antidepressants (Anafranil) for >10 years of age

   Selective serotonin reuptake inhibitors
   Fluoxetine (Prozac) for >7 years of age
   Fluvoxamine (Luvox) for >7 years of age
   Sertraline (Zoloft) for >6 years of age

3) Risperidone (atypical antipsychotics). NOT FDA APPROVED. Research not clear on effectiveness).

4) Other options if there is no response to above-mentioned methods:

   Deep brain stimulation, NOT FDA APPROVED

   Research: POTS

JAMA 2004 October 27;292(16): pp. 1969—76 (access abstract via PubMed).

The study included 112 patients, aged 7—17 years. Their Y-BOCS score was 16 or above.

They were treated for 12 weeks (CBT, sertraline, combination CBT/Med, placebo).

Clinical remission = 10 or less score on Y-BOCS.

Results: Combined therapy better than CBT or sertraline alone. CBT and sertraline equally effective.

Recommendation: Children with OCD should be treated with CBT alone or with a combination of CBT and medication.

RESOURCES (WEBSITES, ETC.)

1. National Institute of Mental Health Resource Center: 1-866-615-6464, nimhinfo@nih.gov
2. Substance Abuse and Mental Health Services Administration (SAMHSA): 1-800-662-4357, Behavioral Health Treatment Locator
3. ABCT Association for Behavioral and Cognitive Therapies: Access ABCT web page For "Fact Sheets" on OCD.

CHAPTER 11

PANDAS/PANS Syndromes: What are They and How are They Diagnosed and Treated

CASE VIGNETTE

Jared is a 9-year old patient who was diagnosed with ADHD, combined type at age 7 years, when his teacher complained that he was "always getting out of his seat, needed constant reminders to do his work, and often had trouble with peers for not playing by the rules on the playground." He was begun on stimulant medication, a daily report card of his behavior was placed into effect with parents and teacher, and he was enrolled in the ADHD "social skills class." All these interventions resulted in improved performance in the classroom, both in getting his work done, as well as listening skills, and in more appropriate and acceptable behavior with his peers.

The current appointment was precipitated by mom's concern regarding his sudden onset of constant throat clearing, almost overnight, and the teacher's writing a note that until his symptom is improved, he would need to stay at home, as the noise was so disruptive in the classroom. Mom says he has always had a "tendency for allergy in the spring," manifested by some throat clearing and nasal congestion, and she thought maybe this was a sudden exacerbation due to the trees in bloom currently. She also says he had a sore throat 2 or 3 weeks ago, with fever, but seemed to recover and was not brought in to the clinic.

"Maybe he has a sinus infection she said. He's had those before and they started with a lot of throat clearing."

She also said that he had "wet his bed twice this week which was highly unusual since he had been dry for years."

Although the terms pediatric autoimmune neuropsychiatric disorders associated with *Streptococcus* (PANDAS) syndrome and pediatric acute-onset neuropsychiatric syndrome (PANS) are known to most pediatricians and child psychiatrists, they are not listed as possible diagnoses in the International Classification of Disease nomenclature. Why is this? It is probably due to several factors, but mostly due to uncertainties regarding the possible cause (or causes) as well as controversy regarding the recommended treatments utilized.

This is not a huge problem in pediatrics, as PANDAS/PANS probably involves only 0.1%—0.2 % of the general pediatric population. But the symptoms associated with these "syndromes" can be very stressful to parents and therefore to the clinicians to whom they reach out for help. So these cases show up at Grand Rounds presentations, physician phone consultations, and even parent support groups. Therefore it seems totally appropriate that this topic be discussed in a guide book for the clinician regarding the mental health issues in childhood and adolescence.

PANDAS SYNDROME

The PANDAS syndrome was first described by a pediatrician, Dr. Susan Swedo (now Chief of the Pediatrics and Developmental Branch at the National Institute of Mental Health [NIMH]), and others who were doing research at NIMH on childhood obsessive-compulsive disorder (OCD). They were impressed by the sudden onset of significant OCD traits in a small number of patients (e.g., over a 24- to 48-h period), much unlike the usual description of parents of children/adolescents with OCD, who describe their child's traits occurring gradually over weeks or months. In some patients, it seemed almost like the OCD or tic symptoms developed overnight.

In the initial article describing PANDAS, Swedo et al.,[1] five characteristics were listed as the diagnostic criteria:

1) Acute onset of OCD and/or a tic disorder.
2) The child was prepubertal (e.g., age 3—12 years).
3) The symptoms followed an episodic course of remission and relapsing, rather than a waxing and waning course.

4) There were accompanying neurologic or behavioral symptoms, e.g., choreiform movements, hyperactivity.

5) Symptom exacerbations seemed to follow group A streptococcal (GAS) infections.

Initially Dr. Swedo and her colleagues chose to confine their research to post-GAS infections, although it seemed apparent that other viral infections, e.g., varicella, could trigger a similar response.

In 2004 the abovementioned characteristics were expanded using the following descriptions:

1) The OCD traits and/or tics had to be severe enough to cause an impairment in the child's or adolescent's ability to perform at a level commensurate to pre-symptom level.

2) The arbitrary age exclusion of onset (<age 12 years) pertained to most children (98%) who become immune to GAS by age 12 years, although occasional cases of PANDAS and/or acute rheumatic fever (also a post-streptococcal phenomenon) are seen in children >12 years of age.

3) The onset should be abrupt, to a 1- to 2-day period, with remitting episodes and exacerbations.

4) Exacerbations must be temporally related to GAS infections, documented by positive throat cultures, and/or a rise in GAS titers, e.g., antistreptolysin O titer test (though some streptococcal infections can be perianal with negative throat cultures). In addition, many children with positive throat cultures and evidence of infection do not develop a rising titer, or a high titer from a recent infection may persist. All these findings may add to the complexity of the diagnostic dilemma.

5) Neurologic abnormalities: Those initially listed were hyperactivity, choreiform movements, and tics.

6) Possible somatic symptom traits were also seen, including urinary frequency, mydriasis.

7) Other potential neuropsychiatric symptoms have been added to the diagnostic criteria:
   - Severe separation anxiety
   - Generalized anxiety, often leading to panic attacks
   - Motoric hyperactivity, abnormal movements, restlessness
   - Sensory abnormalities, e.g., sensitivity to light or sound, visual/auditory hallucinations
   - Difficulty with concentration
   - Urinary frequency, enuresis

- Irritability, labile mood swings, aggression, depression, suicidal ideation
- Developmental regression, infantile speech, poorer handwriting

Age at onset is a factor in how PANDAS presents. Under age 10 years, PANDAS is three times more common in boys than in girls and tends to present with OCD, ADHD, and tics. PANDAS presenting in adolescence is more likely to be in females and associated with anxiety/depression.

PEDIATRIC ACUTE-ONSET NEUROPSYCHIATRIC SYNDROME

PANS, on the other hand, refers to all cases of acute onset of OCD traits that cannot be attributed to a recent acute infection, such as GAS, but might have been triggered by other metabolic or inflammatory causes.

The diagnostic criteria for PANS have been specifically enumerated by Chang et al.[2]:

1) Abrupt onset or recurrence of OCD or restricted eating.

2) Other co-occurring neuropsychiatric symptoms (at least two of the following) of a severe nature and acute onset.
   - Severe anxiety (either new onset or acute severe increase in symptoms)
   - Sensory hypersensitivity, e.g., lights, sounds
   - Tics, motoric hyperactivity, worsening handwriting, choreiform movements
   - Regression in developmental abilities
   - Worsening of school performance
   - Mood alterations including anger/rage, depression
   - Urinary frequency, enuresis
   - Sleep problems

3) Symptoms are not due to a known disorder, e.g., Tourette syndrome, Sydenham chorea.

It is obvious that the PANDAS and PANS guidelines overlap a lot. The main difference is the attribution of PANDAS to recent or recurrent GAS infections. There are other subtle differences between the diagnostic criteria for the two conditions:

1) The criteria for diagnosis of PANS require the acute onset of OCD, but not of a tic disorder, whereas the PANDAS diagnostic criteria usually require both OCD and tics.

2) The PANS diagnostic criteria do not require an etiologic component (but PANDAS requires evidence of recent GAS infection).

DIAGNOSIS OF PANDAS/PANS

How does a clinician diagnose PANDAS/PANS? Swedo et al.[3] have outlined several steps in a very comprehensive workup.

1) Complete medical and psychiatric history
2) Physical examination
3) Laboratory tests (blood, maybe cerebrospinal fluid)
4) Others, e.g., magnetic resonance imaging, electrocardiography, electroencephalography, polysomnography, as indicated
5) Rule out other known diagnoses, e.g., Sydenham chorea, autoimmune encephalitis, systemic lupus, and other CNS disorders. **Remember, the diagnosis of PANS is a diagnosis of exclusion.**
6) Also, can symptoms be due to a chronic OCD, or anxiety disorder? (one difference would be that these conditions tend to wax and wane in severity, whereas PANDAS/PANS are abrupt-onset syndromes and have remissions and acute relapses instead of waxing and waning.)

Most authorities seem to be in reasonable agreement regarding the existence of the PANDAS/PANS conditions. The real controversy seems to be in the lack of clear-cut causes, less so in PANDAS, but even in that diagnosis, there are many inconsistencies in the causes. This is then reflected in the discussion of treatment.

The article by Swedo et al.[3] summarizes a meeting consortium held in May 2014 at the National Institutes of Health (NIH) including a large group of experts from many clinical and research communities, such as pediatrics, child/adolescent psychiatry, immunology, infectious diseases, neurology, microbiology, and rheumatology. Although there was not unanimity of opinion on all aspects, from that auspicious group came a set of "guidelines" that were felt to represent the "best practices" from across the country.

TREATMENT OF PANDAS/PANS

The treatment of PANDAS/PANS was outlined in three separate areas:

1) Symptomatic treatments: These were given primary status or priority to be started immediately after the diagnosis was made:
   - psychotropic medications, e.g., selective serotonin reuptake inhibitors (SSRIs)
   - psychoeducation and behavioral interventions, e.g., cognitive behavior therapy (CBT).

2) Immune therapies: Second level of treatment
   - Antiinflammatory medications (e.g., steroids)
   - Immune-modulating therapies (e.g., immunoglobulin)
3) Antimicrobials
   - Initial course of antibiotics, e.g., for 1 month
   - Long-term prophylaxis
4) In severe life-threatening cases, other more drastic measures are to be considered, e.g., plasmapheresis (by an experienced interdisciplinary team).

How can we pull this all together for the practicing clinician? What recommendations can be made, given the historical ambiguity regarding both the diagnosis and treatment of these symptoms? Several areas of advice would seem to be appropriate.

1) Educate oneself regarding the cardinal traits of PANDAS/PANS, as well as the issues and controversies surrounding the causes and treatment. (To that end a list of references at the end of this article provides a good place to start.)
2) Follow the specific guidelines that have been established by "experts" in making the diagnosis. Utilize these persons, either by phone consultation or 1:1 referral of patients being considered for the diagnosis.
3) Remember the rarity of these specific diagnoses (about 0.1%–0.2% in the general population or one to two per thousand). If one then considers the limited age range (less than 12 years) where most cases occur, it is unlikely that any one primary care clinician would ever see more than one or two patients in a lifetime of practice, compared with the much greater frequency of tic disorders, Tourette syndrome, and OCD (this knowledge should help prevent overdiagnosis).
4) Do not hesitate to provide symptom-relief treatments, e.g., CBT, and medications, e.g., SSRIs, early on, even before PANDAS/PANS is confirmed or rejected, as these treatments are evidence-based therapies for OCD and tic disorders.
5) According to most experts, if PANDAS/PANS is strongly suggested then initiate treatment with an antistreptococcal antibiotic for 30 days. Longer treatment is more controversial.
6) If PANDAS/PANS are confirmed or diagnosed (remember PANS is a diagnosis of exclusion), then strongly consider referral to a "center" for consultation and treatment if secondary or tertiary levels of

treatment are being considered, e.g., intravenous immunoglobulin, chronic steroids, plasmapheresis. Two reasons for this recommendation: one is to avail oneself of an "expert" in the field and another is to make sure the patient is entered into a research database where data is being obtained, e.g., regarding treatment outcomes. Resources include the PANDAS Physicians Network at https://www.pandasppn.org/and the PANDAS Network at http://www.pandasnetwork.org/.

7) Lastly, practice the dictum we all learned in our medical training: "Above all, do no harm."

I am indebted to Dan Coury, MD, FAAP, who was a member of the 2014 PANDAS/PANS Consortium of experts at NIH, who kindly reviewed this article and made some suggestions and additional comments that were incorporated into the manuscript.

REFERENCES

1. Swedo SE, et al. Pediatric Autoimmune Neuropsychiatric Associated with Streptococcal Infection (PANDAS). *Am J Psychiatry.* 1998;155:264–271.
2. Chang K, et al. Pediatric Acute-Onset Neuropsychiatric Syndrome (PANS). *J Child Adolesc Psychopharmacol.* 2015;(1): 3–13. https://doi.org/10.1089/cap.2014.0084.
3. Swedo SE, et al. Overview of treatment of Pediatric Acute-Onset Neuropsychiatric Syndrome (PANS). *J Child Adolesc Psychopharmacol.* 2017;27(7):562–565. https://doi.org/10.1089/cap.2017.0042.

FURTHER READING

1. Swedo SE, et al. Clinical Presentation of pediatric autoimmune neuropsychiatric disorders associated with streptococcal infections in research and community settings. *J Child Adol Psychophaarmacol.* 2015;25:26–30.

CHAPTER 12

Depressive Mood Disorders Secondary or Coexistent With ADHD: Diagnosis and Treatment

MOOD DISORDERS IN ADOLESCENCE: AN OVERVIEW

Mood might best be defined as the emotion a person feels in viewing the life situation around him or her. Is it optimism or sadness? Is it pessimism or hopefulness? The term mood disorder would imply that the emotion was not only negative but also impairing.

A mood disorder denotes a mood that is not normal and not only negative but also impairing.

A) There are several types of mood disorders
   1) Major depressive disorder: A severe depression lasting more than two weeks, with irritability, other significant symptoms, frequent suicidal ideation, or intent (discussed in a following section).
   2) Persistent depressive disorder (dysthymia): Chronic, low-grade depression, lasting 1–2 years or longer (discussed below).
   3) Disruptive mood dysregulation disorder: Diagnosed in children and adolescents <18 years who have chronic irritability and behavior control issues (discussed in Behavior Disorders chapter 14) and more likely to transition into anxiety/depression type picture.
   4) Premenstrual mood disorder: As the name implies.
   5) Mood disorder due to chronic illness, e.g., cancer, diabetes, etc.
   6) Substance abuse–induced mood disorder.
   All of the above mood disorders can be seen in adolescents. It is crucial for the primary care clinician to be alert for mood disorders, which are not rare or even uncommon in adolescents. Various figures regarding the incidence of mood disorders in adolescence appear in the literature, but it appears that 5%–15% incidence rate seems appropriate. However, in specific disorders, e.g., ADHD, the incidence might be higher, perhaps even up to 40%–50% if one looks for persistent depressive disorder (dysthymia).

PEARL: The primary care clinician needs not only to be alert to the incidence of mood disorders but also to the symptoms they produce, and then proactively screen for them, e.g., using the PHQ-9 (depression), along with the SCARED (anxiety) because these two diagnoses often travel together as Siamese twins. (If you screen for one, screen for the other at the same time.)

B) What are possible risk factors for mood disorders?
   1) Family history
   2) Diagnosis of ADHD
   3) History of bullying or being bullied
   4) Parent/friend/relative death (or even a pet)
   5) Separation/Divorce of parents
   6) Chronic health problems, e.g., asthma, diabetes, eating disorder
   7) Learning disability or school failure
   8) Physical defects, abnormalities
   9) Others: physical/mental/sexual abuse, neglect
   10) Pregnancy

C) Other clues/warning signs of mood disorder
   1) Statements such as "I wish I were dead"; or "I might as well kill myself."
   2) Anhedonia: Loss of interest in his/her pleasurable activities.

D) Changes in normal life functions: physical
   1) Eats more, or less; weight loss, or gain.
   2) Sleeps more, or less; nightmares, insomnia.
   3) Psychosomatic complaints.
   4) More active or less active; agitated, restless.
   5) Fatigue, loss of energy.

E) Changes in normal life functions: intellectual
   1) Refuses to do homework.
   2) Skips classes, truant.

3) Fails tests, grades drop.
4) Cannot concentrate, indecisiveness.
5) "Does not care."
6) Changes in executive functioning.

F) Changes in normal life functions: emotional
   1) Cries all the time, or noncommunicative.
   2) Irritability, sadness.
   3) Defeatist attitude, "I can't."
   4) Feeling "worthless," inappropriate, or excessive guilt.
   5) Recurrent thoughts of death.
   6) Suicidal ideation or attempt, e.g., cutting.

G) Changes in normal life functions: social
   1) Quits sports team, choir, or other pleasurable activity.
   2) Refuses to communicate with friends, or changes friends for? Reasons.
   3) Avoids family, stays in bedroom.

H) Other factors
   1) Depression, two to three times more common in females than males.
   2) Suicide risks: Grades 9—12
      17% of adolescents consider it in a given year
      12% of girls and 5% of boys attempt it each year
      (Youth Risk Behavior Study: Center for Disease Prevention and Control)
   3) Most common method in adolescents for suicide is ingestion of pills
   4) Suicides
      • Females are more likely to attempt
      • Males are more likely to succeed (more likely to use guns)

I) Important Pearls for the primary care clinician
   1) Early detection and treatment of mood disorders can reduce severity of symptoms
   2) All the behavior changes that suggest a mood disorder can be due to a substance abuse disorder!
   3) We must have a low threshold of suspicion for mood disorders. (Screen routinely as well as prn symptoms.)
   4) Two important questions to ask if concern raised about depression:
      • "Do you feel a sense of hopelessness about life?"
      • "In the past four weeks, have you considered suicide or self-harm?"
   5) We cannot treat if we do not identify.
   6) Monitoring your adolescent patient's mood obviously requires that you have invested the time and developed the relationship and communication with the adolescent so that you can accurately assess his or her mood.
   7) Substance abuse can cause depression, as can OTC medicines and prescribed medications.
   8) Gay and bisexual/transgender adolescents are at high risk for depression and suicidal ideation/attempt.
   9) History of physical or sexual abuse, or exposure to domestic violence, are risk factors for suicidal attempts!
   PEARL:
   One-half of all adolescents with significant depression are unrecognized as depressed by their families, teachers, or medical caregivers! GO LOOK FOR THEM!
   As primary care clinicians, psychologists, counselors, and special education personnel, we have the knowledge and skills to observe and ask questions that may suggest a mood disorder in our patients.

MAJOR DEPRESSIVE DISORDER
Case Vignette—Major Depressive Disorder
Case 1

A mother brings her 16-year-old daughter, Priscilla, to see you because of her concerns she is depressed. Priscilla has been your patient for several years. You diagnosed her with ADHD, inattentive type, when she entered middle school and had great difficulty getting her assignments on time. Treatment included not only ADHD medications but also a 504 plan for classroom accommodations, a study skills class, and entrance to the "Homework Club" after school. All of this has been very successful in helping Priscilla who is now considered by teachers as a "model student." Mom says in recent weeks things have begun to "slide downhill."

You interview mom and daughter separately, and then together.

Mom lists the following concerns:
1) She stays in her room most of the time.
2) She admits to problems sleeping.
3) She is eating poorly and has lost weight.
4) Her grades are dropping, although she is doing most of her homework.
5) She quits the gymnastic team.
6) She refuses any contact with friends.
7) Further information reveals she was adopted at an age of 4 years from a single mom due to abuse and neglect.
8) Alone, the adolescent confirms she has insomnia, loss of appetite, and weight loss.

9) She also confirms she no longer cares about school or gymnastics.
10) She admits to suicidal ideation, has not made out a plan, but has chosen a method if and when she decides to act upon it.

Major Depressive Disorder

A) The following are the major clinical traits seen in someone with Major Depression, within a 2-week period:
  1) Depressed mood most of the time: Per definition noted in section on "Mood Disorders in Adolescence: An Overview." (In children and adolescents irritability can replace "depressed mood.")
  2) Pronounced lack of interest in most activities.
  3) Marked changes in weight and appetite, increase or decrease.
  4) Sleep disorder, more or less.
  5) Change in activity level: agitation versus lethargy.
  6) Feeling tired, decrease in energy.
  7) Feelings of guilt or lack of worth.
  8) Lack of concentration.
  9) Suicidal ideation, with or without intent or plan.
B) In addition, symptoms must be impairing to some life function, not due to bereavement, other medical conditions, substance abuse, and not accompanied by Mania/Hypomania.
C) Prevalence (per REACH Institute):
  1) Children: 2%. Male/female equal.
  2) Adolescents: 4%–8%. Female:male 2:1.
  3) Higher rates in primary care setting.
    • 50% unrecognized!
D) Clinical course
  1) Some patients rarely have remission (2 months symptom-free); others may have several years free of symptoms between episodes.
  2) Chronicity associated with decreased likelihood of full recovery from symptoms.
  3) **PEARL:** Bipolar disorder may begin as major depressive disorder, particularly those whose symptoms begin in adolescence.
E) Possible precursors
  1) *Individuals with neuroticism* (see life negatively).
  2) *Environmental*, e.g., adverse childhood experiences.
  3) *Family history:* Four times higher incidence in first-degree family members.
  4) *Other nonmood disorders*, e.g., substance abuse, anxiety, borderline personality disorder.
  5) Chronic medical conditions: diabetes, heart disease, asthma, ADHD, etc.

F) Suicide risk
  1) **PEARL:** Always a risk, particularly if there was a previous attempt.
  2) Increased in males, living alone, being single, feelings of hopelessness.
H) Functional consequences
  1) More pain and physical illness.
  2) Decrease in physical and social functioning.
I) Differential diagnosis
  1) Manic/depressive disorder.
  2) Anxiety disorder
  3) Mood disorder due to underlying medical condition.
  4) Depressive disorder due to a drug of abuse, medication, etc.
  5) **PEARL:** ADHD: Shared symptoms of distractibility, low frustration tolerance. (Depression may also be coexistent with the ADHD.)

PERSISTENT DEPRESSIVE DISORDER
Case Vignette—Persistent Depressive Disorder (Dysthymia)
Case 2
You are following a 15-year-old female for ADHD. Things have overall been going reasonably well, but today 1:1 the adolescent appears withdrawn and sad.
1) She admits she has felt sad for months. She attributes her symptoms to being due to this, her first year of high school. She has huge volumes of homework, spends hours every night, barely getting it all finished.
2) She is eating and sleeping poorly. Hardly ever sees her friends except briefly at school.
3) She does not have any hope things will change in the near future.
4) She denies any suicidal ideation or intent, states emphatically, "I could never do that."

Persistent Depressive Disorder (Dysthymia)

A) Persistent depressive disorder (dysthymia) in children and adolescents is the state of feeling chronically sad for a period of 2 years or more. (Irritability can be substituted for the sadness part of the times.)
B) Symptoms of persistent depressive disorder (dysthymia)
  1) Change in appetite: eating more or less
  2) Sleeping more or less
  3) Lethargy
  4) Poor self-image
  5) Difficulty with attention, concentration, or making decisions
  6) Feelings of despair

C) Other requirements for diagnosis: Symptoms must be impairing. Has never been free of symptoms for more than 2 months in a given year, may have some criteria but not enough for diagnosis as Major Depression, does not have symptoms of mania/hypomania, symptoms not due to substance abuse, or a medical condition, or mental health disorder such as psychosis.

I) Diagnostic features
   1) Chronic feeling of "sadness"
   2) Symptom-free periods never longer than 2 months in any given year.

J) Prevalence: 0.5% of population in any given year.

K) Clinical course
   1) Early onset, e.g., childhood, adolescence, early adulthood.
   2) Chronic.
   3) Early onset of symptoms often transition into personality disorder.
   4) Compared with Major Depression, symptoms are more stable and less likely to remit over time.

L) Predisposing factors
   1) *Neuroticism* (see life negatively).
   2) *Environmental*: parental death, separation, or divorce.
   3) Higher incidence in family members.

M) Prognosis
   1) Variable impacts on social and occupational function among individuals.
   2) Outcomes can be worse than major depressive disorder.
   3) Risk of suicide negligent (?) compared with major depressive disorder unless symptoms rise to level of major depressive disorder.

N) Differential diagnosis
   1) Major depressive disorder.
   2) Psychotic disorder.
   3) Depression due to another medical condition.
   4) Substance abuse disorder (or medicine).

PEARL: Always consider screening for substance abuse in a depressed adolescent patient.

DEPRESSION: DIAGNOSIS AND TREATMENT
Diagnosis of Depression

A) History
   (History should be taken from both child/adolescent and parent separately.)
   REMEMBER MENTAL HEALTH CARD!
   1) Review chief complaint
      • Onset, duration, course (constant, episodic?)
      • What makes it worse?
      • What makes it better?
      • Any treatments tried? Better? Worse?
      • Impairment: how, to what degree, etc.
   2) Review of specific symptoms
      (All are commonly seen, although all are not present in every patient.)
      • Appetite increase or decrease? Bulimia
      • Weight loss or gain
      • Insomnia or hypersomnia (increase in sleep)
      • Energy level increase or decrease, fatigue
      • Psychosomatic symptoms: headache, stomachache
      • Feeling worthless, guilt-ridden, shame, low self-esteem
      • Decreased ability to concentrate, school achievement/performance declining
      • Persistent feelings of sadness
      • Problems making decisions
      • Chronic irritability, anger
      • Threatening to run away
      • Feeling hopeless and/or helpless
      • Loss of interest in activities once enjoyed
      • Difficulty with relationships, or lack of interest in friends
      • Feelings of wanting to die
      • Suicidal thoughts or intentions or attempts
   3) Complete medical history (if patient new or unknown to clinician)
      • Growth and development
      • Review of systems
      • Chronic illness
      • Medications, substance usage
      • Other psychiatric conditions, e.g., anxiety
      • History of bullying
      • Sexual history, orientation
   4) School history
      • Like/dislike, hard/easy, boring?
      • History of learning disorders, special education, tutoring
      • Vocational plans/interests/hobbies
   5) Family history
      • Relation with parents, siblings
      • Divorce, blended family
      • Significant deaths (parent, friend, etc.)
      • Genetic: depression, anxiety, bipolar, other psychiatric disorder
      • Suicides
   6) What are the child's best skills?
      • Hobbies, vocational aspirations
   7) Assess suicide risk

B) Physical exam
   • Assess vitals, height, weight (loss)
   • To rule out acute/chronic illness, growth problems

C) Interview 1:1
1) Assess mood: depressed versus sad, etc.
 • Anxious, weepy
 • Posture, eye contact, voice (subdued, vibrant)
2) Perception of problem/symptoms (anger, denial, fear)
3) Review of specific symptoms noted above
4) Discuss peer/family relationships
5) Discuss school problems, concerns
6) Assess communication: lucid, rational, etc.
7) Discuss possible substance abuse; pot, ETOH
8) Discuss suicidal ideation, intent, plan?
D) Laboratory: depends on above
1) If significant weight loss, do screening (anemia, thyroid, blood sugar, etc.)
2) Always consider substance abuse screening in a depressed patient
E) Rating scales
1) PHQ-9 (depression)
2) SCARED (anxiety)
3) Others as indicated, e.g., aggression, BPD (see chapter on Rating Scales), CRAFFT
F) Determine level of Functional Impairment in several domains:
1) Home
2) Social/peers
3) School
4) Sports and other activities

Treatment of Depression

A) Development of treatment plan

1) Assess level of depression (mild, moderate, severe). Used with permission of the GLAD-PC Steering Committee and the REACH Institute Guidelines for Grading Severity of Depression

	Category	Mild	Moderate	Severe
1	Number of symptoms	5–6	[a]	"Most"
2	Severity of symptoms	Mild	[a]	Severe
3	Degree of functional impairment	Mild or no impairment but with substantial and unusual effort	[a]	Clear-cut observable disability

[a] "Moderate" = severity intermediate between mild and severe.

2) Discuss, educate, and counsel patient and family regarding depression and therapy options.
3) Develop a treatment plan with patient and families:
 • Set therapy goals (home, school, peer settings, etc.)
 • Establish a safety plan (suicide prevention). Remove guns, knives, meds, etc.
 • Establish an emergency communication system if symptoms worsen, becomes suicidal, etc.
4) Establish links with appropriate mental health resources in the community.
B) Specific treatment
1) Mild severity: May consider "Active Support and Monitoring"
 • Weekly or biweekly visits (monitoring) Encourage good lifestyle, e.g., nutrition, rest, exercise.
  Not "watch and wait"
 • Eliminate alcohol, pot, etc.
 • May need to work with school to decrease stress, homework, etc.
2) Moderate or severe depression (or complication of substance abuse, etc.)
 • Referral to a mental health clinician for evaluation and treatment (using only evidence-based therapy)
  a) Cognitive behavior therapy (CBT) (see chapter on Anxiety regarding this treatment) or
  b) Interpersonal therapy (1:1 with psychiatrist/psychologist)
 • SSRI medication
 • **PEARL:** Use both behavior therapy and medication in severe depression.
  Note: Treatment for Adolescent Depression Study (TADS).
  (Reference in Section "Hallmark Studies to Read.")
  Large multisite study of adolescent depression, which showed that SSRI treatment was superior to CBT alone, but adding CBT to SSRI gave even better results.
  Certainly, for Severe Depression, combined treatment should be the treatment of choice, and for most, if not all, Moderately Severe Depression as well.

C) Medications FDA approved for use in childhood/adolescent depression
  1) SSRIs are the recommended medications for initial treatment of adolescent depression.
     - Only two SSRI's are FDA approved
       a) Fluoxetine (Prozac) 8–18 years of age
       b) Escitalopram (Lexapro) 12–17 years of age
       c) Sertraline (Zoloft) FDA approved for anxiety treatment but not officially for depression, although commonly used successfully in child/adolescent depression.
  2) Non-SSRI Meds: usually used in special circumstances by child/adolescent psychiatry
     - Tricyclic antidepressants (TCAs)
     - Monoamine oxidase inhibitors (MAOIs)
  3) Dosages

	Starting	Target Range (Daily)	Peak
Fluoxetine (Prozac)	5–10 mg	5–40 mg	4–6 weeks
Sertraline (Zoloft)	25 mg	50–200 mg	4–6 weeks
Escitalopram (Lexapro)	5	5–20	4–6 weeks

  4) Titration
     - "Start low, go slow"
     - Increase to target dose by 4 weeks
  5) If no effect, or inadequate response by 6 weeks, discontinue and try another medication.
  6) Need to taper off SSRIs due to possible withdrawal symptoms, worsening Depression, etc. (Prozac less likely, due to long half-life, to cause rebound symptoms. Unless Prozac dose is excessive, e.g. over 25 mg it can usually be discontinued when new SSRI started.)
  7) How to "cross-taper" to new SSRI
     - Decrease current SSRI by 50%
     - Start new medication at "starting dose"
       PEARL: Do above simultaneously.
  8) Common side effects to SSRI medications:
     Dry mouth
     Constipation
     Diarrhea
     Sweating
     Sleep disturbance
     Sexual dysfunction
     Irritability
     Headache

"Disinhibition" (risk-taking behavior, increased impulsivity)
Agitation or jitteriness
Appetite change
Rashes
More serious side effects to SSRI medications:
Serotonin syndrome: fever, hyperthermia, restlessness, confusion (can be life-threatening)
Hypomania
Suicidality
Akathisia (feeling of motor restlessness, urge to move about, inability to sit still)
Discontinuation syndrome (dizziness, drowsiness, nausea, lethargy, headache)
In all these situations, immediately consult psychiatry regarding how to discontinue medication, how to monitor symptoms, etc.

D) Ongoing management
  1) Monitor treatment goals and outcomes (e.g., weekly for 4–6 weeks or so, then biweekly, then monthly)
     - Assess depression symptoms
     - Assess functioning in home, school, peer groups
  2) Reassess diagnosis and treatment if no improvement is noted after 6-8 weeks
     - Referral to mental health consultant (psychiatry)
  3) Partial response to treatment, both regarding symptoms and/or impairment should trigger a referral to mental health consultant (psychiatry) as well.
  4) Continue to follow patient collaboratively with the mental health consultant regarding roles and responsibilities of each provider.
  5) Rating scales, e.g., PHQ-9, very helpful in monitoring symptoms of depression over ensuing weeks or months.
     Resource: See TADS Study in Hallmark Research Studies Section.

GUIDELINES FOR ADOLESCENT DEPRESSION IN PRIMARY CARE: PARAPHRASED

This document, the result of a large task force of people representing many organizations that impact adolescent care, should be physically present and available in all clinic facilities that deal with adolescent healthcare (physician offices, school clinics, public health, and private agencies, etc.). The Guidelines for Adolescent Depression in Primary Care (GLAD-PC) were first published in 2007 and recently were revised and published in Pediatrics, March 2018. The guidelines can be accessed online through the American Academy of Pediatrics website, www.aap.org, and then using the search engine to find the "GLAD-PC Toolkit."

The following is a paraphrased summary of the newly revised guidelines which include several recommendations in the areas of practice preparation, identification, and surveillance; assessment and diagnosis; initial management; and treatment of adolescent depression. (The GLAD-PC manual, which contains a lot of other information regarding safety precautions in the home, how to monitor the depression symptoms, etc. is being rewritten as this time and will be available at a later date through the American Academy of Pediatrics, www.aap.org. It is highly recommended that any physician/clinician/clinic setting, etc. have a copy of this updated set of GLAD-PC physically available in the clinic setting, for ready access.)

Guidelines for Adolescent Depression in Primary Care Recommendations

A) Practice preparation
  1) Recommendation: Primary care clinicians need to make sure they are trained and qualified to adequately identify, assess, diagnose, and treat adolescents who are depressed.
  2) Recommendation: Primary care clinicians should know about and collaborate with, resources both in the local community as well as state or regional areas, for consultations when necessary to facilitate diagnosis for challenging cases. This may also involve collaboration with other patients and families who have also dealt with adolescent depression.
B) Identification and surveillance
  1) All adolescents (12 years and above) should be routinely screened yearly for depression using a validated screening tool for depression.
  2) Adolescents who have risk factors for depression, including but not limited to the following, should particularly be screened for the development of depression, not only yearly but also whenever indicated by patient symptoms, by using a validated screening tool, e.g., history of prior depression diagnosis, family history of depression, substance abuse, psychosocial problems, trauma, somatic complaints, previous abnormal depressions score on a valid screening, etc.

C) Assessment and diagnosis
  1) Primary care clinicians should evaluate for depression anyone who screens positive on a validated screening tool, anyone with persistent emotional problems, or anyone who seems possibly depressed despite normal scores on screening tools.
  2) Assessment for depression involves interviewing both family members and patient (alone) and must include an assessment of functional impairment in several life areas (school, home, peers, etc.), as well as assessment for other comorbid psychiatric disorders (e.g., anxiety, etc.)
D) Initial management of depression
  1) Clinicians should provide education and counseling regarding depression for both the patient and his or her family including all the options for treatment. Confidentiality should be stressed also.
  2) If the clinician is trained and confident in depression treatment, he or she should discuss and develop with the patient and family a treatment plan which includes goals of treatment in several areas of functioning, such as school, home, social settings, etc.
  3) The treatment plan should include a safety plan, and emergency communication criteria if the patient's symptoms worsen, or deteriorate such as suicidal ideation or intent, possible harm to others, or any other crisis within the patient's environment, especially during the early phase of treatment when such concerns are the greatest.
E) Treatment:
  1) Primary care clinicians should organize their clinics to provide integrated, collaborative care with other mental health personnel including psychiatrist, case managers, and other therapists.
  2) In cases of mild depression, it is reasonable to consider active support and monitoring (NOT WATCH AND WAIT) as an initial treatment rather than evidence-based therapies.
  3) In cases of moderate or severe depression, or if there are other complicating factors, e.g., substance abuse, or other mental health diagnoses, consultation with a mental health specialist should be considered. Subsequently the respective roles of the mental health specialist and the primary care clinician should be carefully

delineated. In addition, the family members should not only confirm these roles but be active team members as well.

4) Primary care clinicians should recommend only evidence-based treatments for depression (e.g., CBT or IPTA [interpersonal therapy], psychotherapies, or medications such as SSRIs) whenever indicated.

5) If medications such as SSRIs are prescribed, primary care clinicians should monitor for adverse side effects.

F) Ongoing management:

1) Patients should be monitored regularly regarding goals and outcomes of treatment, including both symptoms and functional impairment in several life domains.

2) If no improvement in symptoms is noted after 6–8 weeks of treatment, a referral to a mental health consultant should be considered.

3) If only partial improvement in symptoms is seen, despite ruling out such factors as poor compliance, other comorbid conditions should be considered for a mental health consultation.

4) Primary care clinicians should continue to be involved in the depressed adolescent's care even if he or she is being treated by a mental health consultant, so that optimal management is achieved. This may require increased communication between both care providers, as well as careful delineations of the roles and responsibilities of each.

AAP UPDATE ON ADOLESCENT SUICIDE PREVENTION (PUBLISHED JUNE 2016, EDITED)

Case Vignette: You have been following Evelyn, a 17-year-old high school student in 11th grade, with diagnoses of ADHD, inattentive type, and dysthymia. Her ADHD seems adequately controlled by her stimulant medications, and school accommodations per a 504 Plan, e.g., preferential seating, shortened assignments, use of a tape recorder for lectures, and a study skills class where she does her homework with supervision if needed. Her GPA, which was only 1.8 in 9th grade, has risen to 3.0.

Her dysthymia has been of "mild severity," and has been treated by "active support and monitoring," e.g., she is seen every 2–3 weeks in clinic and completes serial PHQ-9 questionnaires. She has been instructed in good health habits regarding sleep, exercise, and nutrition.

Alone, Mom expresses new concerns, e.g., she is not eating as well, complains she feels "tired all the time," and spends most of her time alone in her room.

When seen 1:1 by you, Evelyn looks "depressed," and agrees she feels "life is hopeless." She feels she would be "better off dead," and has contemplated suicide, although she has not developed a plan. Her PHQ-9 scores at 18 today, up from a score of 7 three weeks ago.

A) Facts

1) Suicide is now the second leading cause of death, ages 15–19 years (replaces homicide, which is now at number three)

2) Attempts outnumber successes, 50–100:1

3) Top four methods:
- Suffocation (mostly hanging)
- Guns
- Poisoning (meds, etc.)
- Falling

4) Females are more likely to attempt suicide; males are more likely to succeed in doing so (males are more likely to use guns)

5) Suicide risk is increased in homes with firearms

B) Risk factors for attempting suicide

1) Family history of suicide
2) Drug or alcohol abuse
3) Male sex
4) Sexual identity issues
5) Conflict with parents
6) Problems with school, or absenteeism
7) Bullying, including cyber bullying
8) History of physical or sexual abuse

C) Factors increasing the risk

1) Depression
2) Bipolar disorder
3) Sleep disorder
4) Psychosis
5) Posttraumatic stress disorder
6) Panic attacks
7) History of impulsivity
8) History of aggressiveness
9) Internet usage >5 h/day

D) Red flags!

1) Intent
2) Evidence of a plan
3) Prior attempt (particularly if a lethal method had been utilized), including nonfatal self-harm (see below)
4) Hopelessness, agitation
5) Severe mood disorder

E) Factors possibly lowering risk
  1) Getting along well with parents and peers and at school
  2) Adolescents who practice a religion
F) Advice for pediatricians
  1) Inquire regarding risk factors when taking an adolescent medical history
  2) See adolescents 1:1
  3) Use depression rating scales frequently or even routinely, e.g., PHQ-9
  4) Be aware of myriad symptoms of mood disorders (see previous chapters on Anxiety, Depression, BPD, and Mood Disorders)
  5) Be able to discuss with patient and family the treatment of mood disorders, including both counseling (CBT) and medication (SSRIs)

PEARL: Nonfatal self-harm is a risk factor (27-fold) for suicide, particularly in Native Americans and Alaska Natives within one year of an episode of self-harm, as per a recent study from AHRQ (Agency for Healthcare Research and Quality) reported in Pediatrics, March 2018 online ($n = 32{,}395$ Medicaid patients aged 12–24 years).

Resource: Tool for Assessment of Suicidality in Pediatric Patients.

Adolescent Suicidality Questionnaire (ASQ). Developed by NIMH (National Institute of Mental Health), the questionnaire contains five questions and takes 20 seconds to complete. A "Yes" response to any of the first four questions identified 97% of youth (ages 10–21 years) at risk for suicide.

Available at: https://www.nimh.nih.gov/labs-at-nimh/asq:toolkit-materials/index.shiml.

With links to (1) ASQ Tool; (2) Info Sheet; (3) Suicide Prevention; (4) Resources, etc., it is available in 8 languages!

Important: SHOULD BE ANSWERED WITHOUT THE PARENTS PRESENT!

If screening is positive, patient should receive a Brief Suicide Safety Assessment (BSSA) by an appropriate clinician or counselor, and decide what to do next, e.g., more evaluation, etc. Should also be given the Patient Resource List mentioned above, which includes the following:

National Suicide Prevention Lifeline: 1-800-273-8255.

Crisis Text Line: HOME to 741-741.

Suicide Prevention Resource Center www.sprc.org.

NIMH www.nimh.nih.gov.

Substance Abuse and Mental Health Services Administration www.samhsa.gov.

PEARL: United States Preventive Care Task Force (USPCTF) in January 2016 published in *JAMA* 2016 its guidelines with the following recommendation (edited):

Due to the potential detrimental effects on infants and children, all postpartum women should be screened for maternal depression.

One way to do this is clinically face to face at the time of a postpartum visit (by OB/GYN).

Those of us caring for the infants and children can (should?) utilize a good adult screening tool (when we see the infant) such as:

- PHQ-9 (Patient Health Questionnaire), www.brightfutures.org
- Edinburgh Postnatal Depression Scale (EPDS), www.brightfutures.org

Both tools are available free online. www.brightfutures.org.

PEARL: "Persistent postpartum depression (beyond 6 months) worsens outcomes for children."

Netsi E et al., Dept. of Psychiatry, Oxford University, UK. JAMA Psychiatry. 2018; https://doi.org/10.1001/jamapsychiatry.2017.4265.

Measured child outcomes, behavior problems, leaving school, math, and depression, in 8287 children of 9848 moms. Followed for 11 years after childbirth. Findings: persistent depression doubled risk for behavior disturbances, lowered math scores at age the age of 16 years, increased depression rate at age 18 years. Recommendation: Screen for maternal depression both early and late in first postpartum year.

Some Ways to Help Prevent Suicide in Depressed Adolescents (GLAD-PC). (Used With Permission From the GLAD-PC Guidelines Committee and the REACH Institute)

Some Ways to Help Prevent Suicide in Depressed Adolescents

(Adapted by GLAD-PC with permission from materials prepared by Families for Depression Awareness: http://www.familyaware.org/parentandteenguide.php)

1. **Encourage adolescents and parents to make their homes safe.** In teens ages ten to nineteen, the most common method of suicide is by firearm, followed closely by suffocation (mostly hanging) and poisoning. All guns and other weapons should be removed from the house, or at least locked up. Other potentially harmful items such as ropes, cords, sharp knives, alcohol and other drugs, and poisons should also be removed.

2. **Ask about suicide.** Providers and parents should ask regularly about thoughts of suicide. Providers should remind parents that making these inquiries will not promote the idea of suicide.

3. **Watch for suicidal behavior.** Behaviors to watch for in children and teens include:

- expressing self-destructive thoughts
- drawing morbid or death-related pictures
- using death as a theme during play in young children
- listening to music that centers around death
- playing video games that have a self-destructive theme
- reading books or other publications that focus on death
- watching television programs that center around death
- visiting internet sites that contain death-related content
- giving away possessions

4. **Watch for signs of drinking.** If a child has depression, feels suicidal, and drinks a lot of alcohol, the person is more likely to take his or her life. Parents are usually unaware that their child is drinking. If a child is drinking, the parent will need to discuss this with their child and the clinician.

5. **Develop a suicide emergency plan.** Work with patients and parents to decide how do proceed if a child feels suicidal. It is important to be specific and provide adolescents with accurate names, phone numbers and addresses.

F 1.2

Family Support Action Plan (Depression). (Used With Permission From the GLAD-PC Guidelines Committee and the REACH Institute)

Family Support Action Plan
What a Parent Can Do to Help Their Child/Adolescent

Family Support is a vital component in your child/adolescent's recovery from depression. It makes you a more engaged participant in your child's health care and helps rebuild your child/adolescent's confidence and sense of accomplishment. However, it can also be extremely difficult—after all, when your child/adolescent is depressed, s/he probably doesn't feel like accomplishing anything at all!

To help with Family Support, set goals to help you focus on your child/adolescent's recovery and recognize your child/adolescent's progress. Find things that have helped your child/adolescent in the past—identify goals that are simple and realistic and match your child/adolescent's natural "style" and personality. Work on only one goal at a time.

Adherence to Treatment Plan. Following through on health advice can be difficult when your child/adolescent is down. Your child/adolescent's success will depend on the severity of his/her symptoms, the presence of other health conditions, and your child/adolescent's comfort level in accepting your support. However, your child/adolescent's chances for recovery are excellent if you understand how you and your family naturally prefer to deal with your child/adolescent's health problems. Knowing what barriers are present will help you develop realistic health goals for your child/adolescent. *Example goals:* Remember to give your child/adolescent his/her medications. Participate in counseling. Help your child/adolescent keep appointments.

MY GOAL: _____

Relationships. It may be tempting for your child/adolescent to avoid contact with people when s/he is depressed, or to "shut out" concerned family and friends. Yet, fulfilling relationships will be a significant part of your child/adolescent's recovery and long-term mental health. Understanding your child/adolescent's natural relational style for asking for and accepting help should guide the design of your Family Support plan. *Example goals:* Encourage your child/adolescent to talk with a friend every day. Attend scheduled social functions. Schedule times to talk and "just be" with your child/adolescent.

MY GOAL: _____

Nutrition and Exercise. Often, people who are depressed don't eat a balanced diet or get enough physical exercise—which can make them feel worse. Help your child/adolescent set goals to ensure good nutrition and regular exercise. *Example goals:* Encourage your child/adolescent to drink plenty of water. Eat fruits and vegetables. Avoid alcohol. Take a walk once a day. Go for a bike ride.

MY GOAL: _____

Spirituality and Pleasurable Activities. If spirituality has been an important part of your child/adolescent's life in the past, you should help to include it in your child/adolescent's current routine as well. Also, even though s/he may not feel as motivated, or get the same amount of pleasure as s/he used to, help him/her commit to a fun activity each day. *Example goals:* Recall a happy event. Do a hobby. Listen to music. Attend community or cultural events. Meditate. Worship. Do fun family activities. Take your child/adolescent to a fun place s/he wants to go.

MY GOAL: _____

(Adapted with permission from Intermountain Healthcare)

"Active Monitoring" Not "Watch and Wait" (Depression). (Used With Permission From the GLAD-PC Guidelines Committee and the REACH Institute)

Active Monitoring

Given the tumultuous nature of adolescence, the episodic nature of depression, and the mixed data regarding response to even the most evidence-based treatments, immediate treatment of a new-onset mild to moderate depressive episode may not always be indicated. However, rather than **watchfully waiting** to see if depressed adolescents improve, this guideline advocates **active monitoring** instead. This subtle distinction in word choice is meant to discourage a passive approach and emphasize all of the important things a primary care physician can do BEFORE initiating a formal psychotherapeutic or pharmacological treatment. The following list contains only some of the various ways in which primary care physicians and/or care managers can actively engage with depressed youth while monitoring for changes in their clinical exam:

- Schedule frequent visits (frequency recs to be determined)
- Prescribe regular exercise and leisure activities
- Recommend a peer support group
- Review Self-Management goals
- Follow-up with patients via telephone
- Provide patients and families with educational materials

Education of patients and family members (and -- when indicated and informed consent is obtained -- teachers and/or peers) is a crucial part of active monitoring that can broaden an individuals support network and improve the chances that clinical changes are observed. Please see the parent and adolescent educational materials sections as well as our website (www.gladpc.org) for resources that may be copied for distribution to your own patients and families.

It is important to note that while active monitoring does not have to be continued indefinitely, it should be continued even after individuals improve. If, after a pre-determined amount of time, your patient's depression fails to improve or clinically worsens, an evidence-based treatment is indicated.

BRIEF BEHAVIOR THERAPY

What is "brief behavior therapy" (BBT). I am not sure there is a specific definition currently of BBT, but the current medical literature seems to present it as an attempt to "think out of the box." Because of the current overwhelming need for mental health services, clinicians are designing other ways to do behavior therapy, to see if we can obtain the same or perhaps even better outcomes with using some new ways of doing things. An example would be the article in a previous section about assigning a caseworker to a depressed adolescent, to improve compliance with taking medication, getting to all the counseling appointments, etc. And the results indeed showed improved outcomes from the usual approach of presuming the patient would reliably do all that was requested, e.g., take the medication as directed, make the counseling appointments, and attend all of them, etc.

The background for this discussion is an article recently appeared in the medical literature by Weersing V, et.al. JAMA Psychiatry. 74(6) pp. 571-578. June. 2017.

These researchers studied 186 children, aged 8—16 years, who were randomized equally to two groups: (1) BBT (95 patients), (2) assisted referral to care (ARC) (90 patients).

The BBT group patients received 8—12 weekly sessions of counseling with a masters' level therapist who was conveniently located in the office complex of the primary care clinician.

The ARC group all received personalized referrals to outside masters' level therapists.

Diagnoses of the patients included major depression, dysthymia, generalized anxiety disorder, separation anxiety, social phobia, etc. Excluded from the study were patients with suicidal ideation, substance abuse, PTSD, psychosis, and intellectual disability.

Outcome measures included the clinical global impression and pediatric anxiety rating scale.

Results: The researchers state that the patients receiving BBT showed superior results for treatment of anxiety and depression compared with the ARC group who were referred to outpatient mental healthcare.

Why? Probably the study is not large enough, or the variables are not well enough controlled to really answer that question, although one might speculate that receiving the counseling in the physician's office complex certainly could improve compliance, and therefore improved results.

Probably even more creative ideas will be coming along to help solve our increased needs for treatment resources. Remember "necessity is the mother of invention."

CHAPTER 13

Distinguishing ADHD From Juvenile Bipolar Disorder and Psychosis

BIPOLAR DISORDER: WITH ROBERT KOWATCH, MD, FAACAP

Why is it important to have a chapter on bipolar disorder (BPD) in a book designed for primary care clinicians? Are we expected to be capable of making this diagnosis, choosing an appropriate medication, and monitoring the child's treatment?

In truth the answer is usually "No," but there are some extenuating circumstances that require us to be well informed about diagnosis and management, and in some instances to at least make a tentative diagnosis to be confirmed by a child psychiatrist.

1) Children eventually diagnosed with juvenile BPD are already in our practice, possibly being followed up by us for another diagnosis, often ADHD or depression. Recognizing the overlapping of symptoms and the presentation of new signs and symptoms should alert us to a possible change in diagnosis, and especially to a need for a major change in therapy.

2) Many conditions we diagnose and follow, such as ADHD, oppositional defiant disorder (ODD), conduct disorder (CD), and major depressive disorder, cannot only be "look-alikes" of BPD, but often are comorbid disorders of the BPD itself. So this risk pool of patients need diligent and close monitoring for a change to a bipolar pattern.

3) The medicines used to treat BPD in children and adolescents have significant side effects, which require close monitoring. We primary care clinicians need to be the guardians of that monitoring to assure that it is done properly and the child's physical health is protected.

4) We will probably continue the responsibility of refilling the medications for the other comorbid disorders (e.g., ADHD) and may need to coordinate refills of the BPD medications as well. Hence the need for us to be fully informed regarding this diagnosis and treatment.

So let us look at what is known about BPD in children and adolescents.

Prevalence: About 1%–3%; mean, ~1.5% (depending on the study).

- Peak age, 15–19 years
- A pediatric panel of 2000 patients (assume 800 adolescents) could have ~8–10 patients with BPD (compared with about 200 patients with ADHD).
- These data are from adolescents because incidence in children with BPD is not well known.
- Higher incidences in females of all ages.
- If one parent is already diagnosed with BPD, the odds are increased by five times.

PEARL: Despite these, negative family history does not rule out BPD and a positive family history does not rule it in.

Many patients may present with the chief complaint of "mood swings" but few are bipolar. The following discusses two short case histories of patients with "mood swings": one with BPD and another without BPD.

CASE 1

Elliot is a 13 y/o male with a history of ADHD brought in by his single mother because of his "mood swings." He was treated in the past with Adderall XR, 10 mg, po q AM for ADHD. His mother reports that this medication has helped his school grades but not his "attitude." She reports that anytime she asks him to do anything at home he throws a "fit" and screams at her, "Leave me alone." He has few friends and he spends most of his free time playing Doom with them online. His mother reports that he has been like this "since he was little" and that his attitude has caused him problems at school and with other adults. His mood swings are "constant," three to four times/ day, last 15–20 min, and are relieved "when he gets his way." His appetite and sleep are good and his grades in school "have always been "mediocre." He denies any anxiety symptoms and his biologic father left the family after he was born.

CASE 2

Penny is a 15 y/o female whom you have followed up since childhood for nonspecific mood and anxiety problems. When she was 3 years old, she developed marked separation anxiety that resolved with school and parental support after she entered first grade. In third grade, she became depressed for about 3 months during the winter and she responded to therapy with a local Masters in Social Work (MSW). For the past several weeks, she has been waking up at 3 a.m., making copious notes about what her plans for the future and practicing her violin. Her mother reports that she has" become "obsessed with global warming and will talk rapidly for hours about her plans to fix this. Her teachers have noted that she has been much more "assertive" in class, asking a lot more questions and at times going off on tangents. Her mother reports that her mood is a lot more "up," she has more energy and has been engaging in multiple projects at school and home. There is no suspicion of any substance abuse. Her mother has a history of anxiety and her father was an alcoholic but is now sober. The family denies any changes or stressors in their life.

SYMPTOMS OF BIPOLAR DISORDER

"Mood swings" are common and nonspecific, whereas "mood cycles" are characteristic of children and adolescents with BPD. Mood cycles are pronounced shifts in mood and energy from one extreme to another. An example of this would be a child who wakes up with extreme silliness, high energy, and intrusive behavior that persists for several hours, then several hours later becomes sad, depressed, and suicidal with no precipitant for either mood cycle.

Pediatric patients with BPD will also exhibit other symptoms of mania during these mood-cycling periods.
- **Elevated or expansive mood:** The patient will often have a mood that is inappropriately giddy, silly, elated, or euphoric. Often this mood will be present without any reason and will last for several hours. It may be distinguished from a transient cheerful mood by the intensity and duration of the episode.
- **Irritable mood:** The child may become markedly belligerent or irritated with intense outbursts of anger, two to three times/day for several hours at a time. An adolescent may appear extremely oppositional, belligerent, or hostile with their parents and other people.

- **Grandiosity or inflated self-esteem:** This can potentially be confused with brief childhood fantasies of increased capability. Typically, true grandiosity can be seen as assertions of great competency in all areas of life, which usually cannot be altered by contrary external evidence. Occasionally, this may be bizarre and include delusions of "superpowers." During a manic episode a child will not only assert that he/she can fly but also jump off the garage roof to prove it.
- **Decreased need for sleep:** The child may only require 4–5 h/night of sleep over the period of a manic episode without a subjective feeling of fatigue or evidence of tiredness. Substance use should be considered in this differential, particularly for adolescents.
- **Increased talkativeness:** The child or adolescent has a sustained period of uncharacteristically increased speech. Lack of inhibition to social norms may lead them to blurt out answers during class or repeatedly be disciplined for talking to peers in class. Speech is typically very rapid and pressured to the point where it may be continuous and seems to jump between loosely related subjects.
- **Flight of ideas or racing thoughts:** The child or adolescent may report a subjective feeling that their thoughts are moving so rapidly that their speech cannot keep up. Often this is differentiated from rapid speech by the degree of rapidity with which the patient may express loosely related subjects, which may seem completely unrelated to the listener.
- **Distractibility, short attention span:** During the episode the child or adolescent may report that it is impossible to pay attention to class or other outside events because of the rapidly changing focus of their thoughts. This symptom must be carefully distinguished from the distractibility and inattention of ADHD, which typically is a more fixed and long-standing pattern rather than a brief episodic phenomenon in a manic or hypomanic episode.
- **Increase in goal-directed activities:** During a milder episode the child or adolescent may be capable of accomplishing a great deal of work. However, episodes that are more severe manifest as an individual starts numerous ambitious projects that he/she is unable to complete later.
- **Excessive risk-taking activities:** The child or adolescent may become involved in forbidden

pleasurable activities that have a high risk for adverse consequences. This may appear as hypersexual behavior, frequent fighting, increased recklessness, use of drugs and alcohol, shopping sprees, or reckless driving.

There are two types of bipolar episodes: manic and hypomanic.

MANIC EPISODE
A distinct period of expansive and/or irritable mood that lasts for at least a week.
1) Symptom traits of a manic episode
   - Grandiosity or heightened self-esteem
   - Decreased sleep requirement
   - Hypertalkative
   - Racing thoughts or ideas
   - Distractibility
   - Increased activity level or agitation
   - Participation in pleasurable activities that have possible painful outcomes, e.g., shopping sprees, sexual activity
2) Results in impairment of social and occupational functioning
3) Symptoms are not due to substance abuse, medication, or another medical disorder

HYPOMANIC EPISODE
A distinct period of elevated and/or irritable mood that persists for at least 4 days.
1) Symptom traits of a hypomanic episode
   - Grandiosity or heightened self-esteem
   - Decreased sleep requirement
   - Hypertalkative
   - Racing thoughts or ideas
   - Distractibility
   - Increased activity level or agitation
   - Participation in pleasurable activities that have possible painful outcomes, e.g., shopping sprees, sexual activity
2) Obvious change in the person's normal functioning, which is observed by others
3) Mood and behavior changes are obvious to others
4) No significant impairment in social or occupational functioning
5) Symptoms are not due to substance abuse, medication, or another medical disorder
6) Does not cause a marked impairment in occupational or social functioning or necessitate hospitalization

Manic Versus Hypomanic Episodes

	Manic	Hypomanic
Symptom traits (same symptoms for both types)	Same	Same
Increase in energy and activity	Yes	Yes
Increased elevation in mood/irritability	Yes	Yes
Marked impairment in social/occupational functioning	Yes	No
Requires hospitalization	Usual/often	No
Duration	7 days (or less if hospitalized)	4 days

ADHD Versus Bipolar Disorder: Symptoms Shared

	ADHD	Bipolar
Irritability	Yes	Yes
Short attention	Inattention	More "flight of ideas"
Sleep disturbance	Insomnia	Decreased need for sleep
Symptom duration	Persistent Continuous	Episodic

PEARL: The best discrimination between BPD and ADHD in children and adolescents is the episodes of elation, grandiosity, flight of ideas, racing thoughts, decreased need for sleep, and hypersexuality. These are common in BPD, but rare in ADHD.

PEARL: Usually a manic episode is required to make/confirm the diagnosis of BPD, or at least a "clear history of an episode that is different from the child's normal self."

PEARL: BPD can present initially as depression in adolescents, which is usually sudden and pronounced.

DIAGNOSIS OF BIPOLAR DISORDER (STEPS REQUIRED)
1) Medical history
   As with all mental health conditions obtain information on all domains of the child's life, particularly family history (first- and second-level relatives). SEE MENTAL HEALTH CARD in Chapter 9.
   - Explore whether symptoms are continual/persistent versus episodic
2) Physical examination (see comments in chapters 3, 10, 12, and 14.)

3) 1:1 Interview (see comments in previous chapters)
4) Rule out substance abuse particularly in adolescents
   • Symptoms may mimic BPD or overlap
5) Rating scales (possible usage)
   • Child Behavior Checklist: Screening for ADHD/ODD/anxiety, not specific for BPD
   • Vanderbilt (ADHD)
   • Young Mania Rating Scale: A manic severity scale, not diagnostic or specific
6) Look for coexisting conditions
   • ADHD: Negative behaviors usually impulsive
   • ODD: Negative behaviors often aggressive
   • CD: Negative behaviors are usually planned, goal-oriented, and calculated

   PEARL: In BPD, negative behaviors are mostly due to grandiosity and poor judgment.
7) Laboratory tests
   • Toxicologic screening for suspected substance abuse
   • Metabolic laboratory tests: Fasting glucose, liver functions, cholesterol/free fatty acids (baseline, for use of atypical antipsychotic medications [see chapter 16 on Atypical Antipsychotic Medications.])
8) Consult a mental health specialist (child psychologist or child psychiatrist) for definitive diagnosis

Treatment of Juvenile Bipolar Disorder

(This is rarely done by primary care clinician, unless in coordination with child psychiatry.)
1) Crisis intervention, as needed
2) Ongoing psychiatry follow-up
3) Family/patient ongoing counseling
4) CBT or dialectic behavior therapy

MEDICATIONS

The atypical antipsychotics are used as the first-line treatment because there are multiple large, well-designed, placebo-controlled studies that have demonstrated the efficacy of atypical antipsychotics in children and adolescents with BPD. The following medications (except ZIPRASIDONE) are approved by the FDA for the treatment of manic symptoms in children and adolescents:

• ARIPIPRAZOLE (ABILIFY): FDA-indicated medication used to treat the symptoms of acute mania or mixed episodes associated with bipolar I disorder in children and adolescents aged 10–17 years. Abilify is also approved to help prevent reoccurrence of BPD in children and adolescents, as well as adults.
• OLANZAPINE (ZYPREXA): Indicated by the FDA for adolescents with mania as a second-line treatment agent because of the metabolic effects.

• QUETIAPINE (SEROQUEL): FDA indicated to treat the acute manic symptoms of BPD in children and adolescents.
• ZIPRASIDONE (GEODON, ZELDOX): FDA indicated to treat the manic symptoms of BPD in adults. Ziprasidone, however, does not have an FDA indication to treat children or adolescents with BPD.
• ASENAPINE/SAPHRIS: Indicated as monotherapy for the acute treatment of manic or mixed episodes associated with bipolar I disorder in pediatric patients (ages 10–17 years).
• RISPERIDONE: Has the most amount of research data compare with other atypical antipsychotic medications.

Atypical Antipsychotic	Start at (mg/day)	Target Dose (mg/day)	Monitor	Watch Out for
Risperidone	0.25 –0.50	1–3	Weight/height/BMI	EPS/TD
Aripiprazole	2.5–5	5–20	Weight/height/BMI	EPS
Quetiapine	50 –100	300–600	Weight/height/BMI	
Ziprasidone	20–40	80–160	Weight/height/BMI/ECG	Take with food, assess cardiac risk factors
Olanzapine	5	5–20	Weight/height/BMI	Choles/FAs
Asenapine (sublingual)	5	5–20	Weight/height/BMI	Choles/FAs

BMI, body mass index; *EPS*, extrapyramidal syndrome; *TD*, tardive dyskinesia; *Choles/FAs*, Cholesterol/Fatty Acids.

OLDER MOOD STABILIZERS

Lithium is an older mood stabilizer with a moderate effect size in children and adolescents that is sometimes used as in combination with atypical antipsychotics. Lithium is indicated by FDA for the treatment of acute mania and BPD in adolescents (ages 12–18 years). However, lithium may cause renal, hematologic, thyroid, and other endocrinal changes that must be monitored. Common side effects of lithium that may be particularly problematic for children and adolescents include nausea, polyuria, polydipsia, tremor, acne, and weight gain.

Valproate in its various forms (sodium divalproex) was used for many years to treat mania in children and adolescents. But a large controlled trial of sodium divalproex in children and adolescents with mania showed negative results, and this agent is now used more like lithium as an augmenting agent with an atypical antipsychotic. Common side effects of valproate in children and adolescents include nausea, increased appetite, weight gain, sedation, thrombocytopenia (low blood platelet count), transient hair loss, and tremor.

PSYCHOSIS: WITH ROBERT KOWATCH, MD, FAACAP

Case Vignette: Psychosis

A 16-year-old Middle Eastern male, whose family immigrated to the United States when the child was 4 years

Mood Stabilizer	Start at (mg/kg per day)	Target Serum Level (mg/mL)	Monitor	Watch Out for
Lithium	25−30	0.8−1.2	Renal/thyroid function	Dehydration → toxicity
Valproate	15−20	85−110	Liver/pancreas/platelets	Polycystic ovary syndrome, hyperammonemia
Carbamazepine	15−20	7−10	WBC/platelets	Cytochrome P450 interactions

Old: Lithium, valproate, and carbamazepine.

New: Lamotrigine, etc. (database trial was negative in pediatric BPD).

PEARL for lithium: A primary care clinician needs to know the side effects and to monitor blood levels, baseline laboratory values, target dose, etc. even if primarily followed by child psychiatry.

REFERENCES

Shain, B. et al. Collaborative role of the pediatrician in the diagnosis and management of bipolar disorder in adolescents. *Pediatrics.* 2012;130:e1725−e1742.

Correll, C. MD. Antipsychotic use in children and adolescents: minimizing adverse effects to maximize outcomes. *J Am Acad Child Adolesc Psychiatry.* January 2008;47:1.

Baum R, Kowatch R. Is it ADHD or bipolar disorder? *Curr Psychiatr.* 2014;13(7).

New FDA medication approved for BPD in children and adolescents (March 2018).

Name: Lurasidone (Latuda), Sunovion Pharmaceuticals.

Approved for treatment of major depressive episodes associated with bipolar I disorder in children and adolescents aged 10−17 years. This is a serotonin-dopamine antagonist already approved for treatment of adults with bipolar depression as monotherapy, and as adjunctive therapy with lithium or valproate, and for the treatment of schizophrenia in adults and children aged 13−17 years. Dosage range is 20−80 mg/day. Most common side effects are nausea, weight gain, and insomnia. It is available in 20, 40, 60, 80, and 120 mg doses. Its efficacy in the treatment of mania in BPD has not been established.

old, is brought into your clinic. His parents state that in the past few days he has seemed "agitated," pacing the floor, rarely sitting down. They wonder whether he is "on drugs" because he is having "questionable friends." But they deny that there have been any prior signs or symptoms of substance abuse. Overall, they say, he is an average student described as "bright" by his teachers, who feel he is "not working up to his potential," e.g., sometimes he forgets to do his homework, forgets to turn it in on time, or does not bring the right book home to do his homework. Parents consulted a specialist who felt he had ADHD and "wanted to give him medicine," which they were against, and decided to try some other techniques suggested by the school counselor, e.g., hiring a homework tutor and enrolling him in a study skills class, along with attending homework club after school. They also purchased an extra set of books to keep at home. All of these techniques have been somewhat helpful so at the present time they feel they are not in favor of a medication trial unless things worsened.

His medical history is otherwise unremarkable.

They also comment that a family relative in Iraq was placed in a "mental hospital," but they are unsure about the reason.

Alone, the adolescent does indeed appear agitated, talking rapidly with poor eye contact. He says he recently watched a news program about atrocities being committed overseas, and he is "worried" about the plight of his cousins in Iraq. He also states he has "heard a voice repeatedly telling him to go and help them."

Psychosis in Children and Adolescents

The purpose of this brief section, as in the previous discussion on BPD in children and adolescents, is not to make pediatricians into "mini child psychiatrists," to be comfortable in diagnosis and management of psychosis. Overall, in a general pediatric setting seeing a patient with this condition will be uncommon, more so in the younger child than an adolescent. But as psychosis may present as an acute emergency, we need to know the signs and symptoms to facilitate prompt diagnosis and treatment.

Definition: "Severely disrupted thought and behavior resulting in loss of developmentally appropriate reality testing." (used with permission from The REACH Institute.)

Psychosis can be manifested in several different ways including delusions, hallucinations, disorganized thoughts, abnormal motor behavior, and negative symptoms.

1) **Delusions:** There are several types:
   a) Persecutory: Fear of being harmed by someone or something.
   b) Referential: Feeling that comments or actions by others are directed to oneself.
   c) Grandiose: When one believes he or she is truly exceptional (e.g., beauty, intelligence, gifted).
   d) Erotomanic: Believing incorrectly that someone is in love with him or her.
   e) Nihilistic: Belief that a major disaster is about to occur.
   f) Somatic: Preoccupation with one's body.

   Delusions may at times be bizarre or resemble strongly held beliefs and be hard to assess.

2) **Hallucinations:** Disorders of perception, not due to any actual sensory stimulus.
   a) Auditory: Most common. Hearing voices distinct from one's own thoughts.
   b) Visual: More common in young children. Seeing imaginary objects.

3) **Disorganized thinking (speech)**
   a) Changing topics frequently.
   b) Answering questions with unrelated comments.
   c) Rapid or nonsensical speech that impairs communication.

4) **Grossly disorganized or abnormal motor behavior**
   a) Silliness, agitation
   b) Catatonia, mutism
   c) Purposeless or stereotypic movements
   d) Echoing

5) **Negative symptoms**, e.g., diminished facial expression, no eye contact, no speech intonation.

   Also includes *avolition* (decreased participation in work or school activities) and *anhedonia* (decreased ability to experience pleasure).

6) **Symptoms that may seem psychotic in children (but are not!):**
   • Illusions: "A distortion of the senses." Most common is optical illusion, "visually perceived objects and images that differ from reality."
   • Imaginary friends (age inappropriate).
   • Fantasy, in the young, cognitively delayed, or language-delayed child.

Differential Diagnosis of Psychosis

Medical conditions associated with possible secondary psychotic symptoms:
1) CNS infections (e.g., encephalitis)
2) Seizure disorders
3) Delirium (e.g., due to fever, infections). An acutely disturbed state of mind that occurs in fever, intoxication, and other disorders and is characterized by restlessness, illusions, and incoherence of thought and speech.
4) CNS neoplasms
5) Endocrine disorders (e.g., thyrotoxicosis)
6) Genetic syndromes
7) Autoimmune disorders
8) Medications
   • Stimulants, hypnotics, sedatives, anxiolytics
   • Over-the-counter medications (e.g., dextromethorphan; abovementioned symptoms due to medications usually resolve within 30 days of stopping medications)
9) Substance abuse (e.g., mushrooms, inhalants, lysergic acid diethylamide, alcohol, cannabis, cocaine), bath salts

PEARL: In a young child with symptoms of psychosis do a good medical workup to rule out the organic cause, with special emphasis on the infections, CNS lesions, side effects to medications, and toxins.

In adolescents, in addition to abovementioned, rule out substance abuse, alcohol, cannabis, or other street drugs.

Psychiatric Conditions Associated with Psychosis

1) Schizophrenia: Rare, about 1% of population, usually showing up in adolescence
2) BPD
3) Major depressive disorder
5) Brief psychotic disorder, e.g., symptoms remit within 30 days
6) Social anxiety disorder

Treatment

1) Psychiatric consultation
2) If urgent, patient is a danger to self or others, referral to hospital emergency room
3) FDA-approved medications (see chapter 16 on Atypical Antipsychotic Medications regarding dosing, side effects, monitoring, etc.)

REFERENCE

Sidhu K, Dickey T. Hallucinations in children: diagnostic and treatment strategies. *Curr Psychiatr.* 2010;9(10).

CHAPTER 14

Behavior Disorders Associated or Coexistent With ADHD

OPPOSITIONAL DEFIANT DISORDER

Case Vignette—ADHD, Oppositional Defiant Disorder

Joey has "always been difficult," says his mom. "He never outgrew being a "terrible two." He is constantly "on the go," won't stay in his seat at school, defies the teacher, says he "doesn't have to do what she says." Joey currently is just starting first grade and is 6.5 years old.

What makes his behavior so difficult to understand, parents say, is that "some days he can just be an angel." But then if provoked, or even when not provoked, he can "fly off the handle," yell and scream and may kick or hit his siblings.

Peers at school stay away from him because of his outbursts, often when he does not get his way during recess games.

Oppositional defiant disorder (ODD) is a behavior disorder manifested by symptom traits of defiance, argumentativeness, and vindictiveness. It is more common in boys and has a prevalence rate of about 3% in the general population. However, according to some studies, the incidence may be as high as 50% in males with ADHD. The symptoms listed commonly appear in the preschool years and may eventually develop into conduct disorder (CD; see later discussion), which involves more antisocial behaviors. Even if CD is not eventually the outcome, ODD often manifests itself in adult life with adjustment issues, impulse control problems, substance abuse, anxiety, depression, and resistance toward authority.

The major signs and symptoms of ODD are
1) chronic angry mood,
2) temper outbursts,
3) resentfulness,
4) argumentative, particularly toward authority figures,
5) refusal or defiance of rules or commands,
6) annoys those around him/her,
7) blames others and refuses sense of responsibility,
8) vindictive.

The behaviors must be impairing to some area of the child's life, such as school or home. The behaviors cannot be secondary to another diagnosis, such as autistic spectrum or psychosis.

Severity is graded from mild (symptoms in one setting) to severe (symptoms in three or more settings).

The risk factors for ODD include the following:
1) Poverty, neglect, history of physical, mental, or sexual abuse
2) Poor, inadequate, or hostile parenting
3) Learning and/or language disabilities
4) Specific diagnoses, e.g., ADHD, as mentioned earlier

Etiology

Most studies do not show genetic or neurobiological markers of ODD. A definitive cause has not been demonstrated.

Treatment

Several treatments will reduce ODD symptoms and are commonly used simultaneously.
1) Parent training in use of behavior-modification techniques, reward for positive behaviors, consequence systems for negative behaviors, time-outs, token economies, etc. Parent training is most effective with 1:1 guidance from a counselor or a series of small-group "intensive" classes, rather than attending one parenting class or just reading a book. (The American Academy of Pediatrics has a small handbook explaining these techniques, available at www.aap.org, which can also be helpful, although not adequate for training of parents in and of itself.)
2) Contingency management: It is "the use of certain techniques, e.g., rewards/consequences to modify behavior response. It involves "on-the-job training" for the child. This might occur in a controlled environment, such as a special school, behavior classroom, summer program, etc.

All these environments require close monitoring in a setting with high adult-to-child ratio so that misbehavior results in an immediate intervention.

PEARL: "Anger management classes" usually do not help much (e.g., the school counselor gets a small group of boys with ODD together for a weekly "anger class").

This is usually a discussion format of how to control their behavior. However, children with ODD, particularly those with ADHD, cognitively know their behavior is wrong, so what they need are behavior interventions to enforce good behavior.

The 1-2-3 magic program, designed by Tom Phelan, PhD, can be a very helpful technique for parents. (One helpful approach is to have copies of the video available to "loan" to parents to help them master the 1-2-3 technique.) Basically 1-2-3 magic is based on the concepts of gradual warning for inappropriate behavior, with the third warning resulting in an intervention. Like "3 strikes and you're out!" (in baseball).

Private schools and summer day camp programs, specially designed for children with problems, can be very helpful but are expensive because of the need for a high adult-to-child ratio for immediate response to a misbehavior.

Many typical summer programs, although excellent and designed for the usual child, cannot provide the type of immediate intervention that will alter the behavior of a child with ODD, mostly because of a low staff-to-child ratio.

3) Medication: They are very important in the child/adolescent with ADHD. Use stimulant medications to the highest dose possible before adding a second medication (e.g., atypical antipsychotic; see following discussion).

PEARL: ODD behavior in children and adolescents with ADHD usually requires higher doses of stimulant medicine to control than what it takes to control ADHD symptoms alone.

4) **Atypical antipsychotics** (e.g., risperidone): Use in addition to a maximum dose of stimulant if needed for uncontrolled ODD behavior in a child with ADHD. They can be very effective. (However, remember that risperidone, although widely used for behavior control mostly by child psychiatrists, is "off-label" for use in this way; so are all atypical antipsychotic medications.) Before prescribing an atypical antipsychotic medication, the clinician must carefully assess the risk/benefit of the severity of the behavior versus the potential severe side effects of the antipsychotic medication. MAKE SURE THAT EVIDENCE-BASED ADHD TREATMENT (FDA-approved ADHD medications and behavior

therapy) HAS BEEN MAXIMIZED BEFORE USING ATYPICAL ANTIPSYCHOTIC MEDICATIONS FOR BEHAVIOR CONTROL IN A CHILD WITH ADHD.

(see chapter 13 re; the use of atypical antipsychotic medications in a non-ADHD child.)

CONDUCT DISORDER
Case Vignette—Conduct Disorder
Jeff was diagnosed with ADHD, combined type, in second grade. Symptoms at that time included marked hyperactivity, impulsivity, and inattention. He took ADHD medication for a few months and did much better. However, parents became alarmed because of decrease in appetite and weight loss. So the medication was discontinued. As school became intolerable because of behavior outbursts, he was homeschooled for the next 3 years.

Recently, his parents were divorced, and mom had to return to the workforce, so Jeff entered sixth grade in a public school. He recently was expelled because of "fighting on the school ground."

Mom is "beside herself" because of multiple behavior concerns recently. For example, he was picked up by the police for shoplifting, he stays out late at night against parent house rules, and he has skipped several days at school. When asked where he was, he says "nowhere." Mom feels he is "angry about the divorce," especially because he rarely sees his dad.

CD is the term used to describe persons who are aggressive toward people or animals or are destructive to property. Its frequent precursor is ODD. If CD traits continue past the age of 18 years then the person should be labeled as having antisocial personality disorder.

The following is a list (not complete) of the types of behaviors that endorse a child/adolescent for the diagnosis of CD:

1) Arson
2) Destroying others' property
3) Lying (to get something)
4) Stealing (e.g., shoplifting)
5) Burglary (break and entering)
6) Running away from home
7) Truancy from school at <13 years of age
8) Being cruel to people or animals
9) Rape
10) Fighting (initiating)
11) Bullying
12) Coercion (physical, mental, sexual)
13) Extortion
14) Using a weapon (knife, gun, club, etc.)

(In other words an antisocial behavior that results in harm to other persons, animals, property, etc.)

Other Diagnostic Criteria

1 *The abovementioned behaviors resulting in impairment in social and academic functioning.*
2 *After age 18 years, if behaviors persist, label as antisocial personality disorder.*

Other Characteristics

1) Incidence: About 4% in general population
   - 20% or so in ADHD population, mostly from hyperactive-impulsive type
   - Men > women
2) Higher rate of substance abuse
3) Higher incidence of suicidal ideation and attempt
4) May begin in early childhood, usually peaks during mid-adolescence
5) ODD is a frequent precursor
6) Majority of cases remit by adulthood
7) Early childhood onset has poorest prognosis
8) Female patients present more with lying, running away, truancy, substance abuse, and prostitution

Risk Factors

1) Lower than average IQ
2) "Difficult temperament" as infant
3) Parental rejection and neglect, harsh discipline, dysfunctional family
4) Physical/sexual abuse
5) Exposure to violence
6) Delinquent peer group
7) Genetics—increased risk if parent or sibling has/had CD (neuroimaging is not diagnostic)
8) ADHD, ODD
9) Mood disorders (anxiety, depression)
10) Specific learning disorders and/or academic failure

Treatment

1) Counseling: Parent versus family versus child
2) Individual psychotherapy (e.g., sexual abuse)
3) Group therapy versus cognitive behavior therapy (anxiety, depression, etc.)
4) Residential placement (ranch, private military school, etc.)
5) Tutor/remediate academic deficiencies
6) Medication
   - None is specific for CD
   - Treat underlying conditions (ADHD, anxiety, depression, etc.) with specific medications (stimulants, selective serotonin reuptake inhibitors (SSRIs), etc.)
   - Atypical antipsychotics (see following section in this chapter 14 re: the Aggressive child.)
7) Substance abuse rehabilitation treatment

THE AGGRESSIVE CHILD: WITH ROBERT KOWATCH, MD, FAACAP

Case Vignette—The Aggressive Child

Ethan is an 8-year-old child recently diagnosed with ADHD, combined type. He is on treatment with Concerta and had a great response for his hyperactivity and inattention. Current concerns, however, are that despite his improved ADHD behavior on medication, he still retains his aggressive traits.

For example, while waiting in line for school assembly, he was accidentally pushed by a peer so he "hauled off and slugged him." Peers have stopped playing with him at recess because he always wants to be in charge and, when they refuse, he "slugs them." At home, his 6-year-old brother is "afraid of him" because he repeatedly takes the child's toys away from him.

He was recently expelled from school because of a temper tantrum and when restrained, he kicked the teacher.

The Aggressive Child

Goal: As primary care clinicians, we need to know how to differentiate the types of aggression, the underlying causes or risk factors associated with aggressive behavior, and the treatments used to treat, minimize, and control aggression in children and adolescents.

It is not presumed that a primary care clinician will be able to handle all, or even most, aggressive patients seen in a clinic. However, many forms of less than moderate to severe aggression, particularly when seen in patients with known diagnoses such as ADHD, can be readily managed if the general principles of therapy are known to the clinician.

It is important to know that aggressive behavior is the primary reason for referrals to child psychiatry, and the primary care clinician who sees patients with ADHD and/or aggressive behavior needs to have open communication and ready access to a psychiatric resource.

Types of aggressive behavior

There are several recognizable types of aggressive behavior depending on the provocation, the degree of response, and the duration of the response.

1) Impulsive or reactive type (e.g., ADHD, ODD)
   - Not provoked
   - Often in response to a threat
   - Usually brief
   - Not goal oriented
2) Premeditated (e.g., CD)
   - planned and executed
3) Hyperarousal type (e.g., anxiety, obsessive-compulsive disorder, posttraumatic stress disorder)
   - Secondary to feeling anxious or overwhelmed
4) Maladaptive type
   - Chronic
   - More intensive, out of proportion to environment
5) Cognitive type (e.g., psychosis)
   - Due to delusions
   - Impairment of reasoning

   PEARL: These types may be seen in combination and in overlapping risk factors.

Risk factors for aggression in childhood

1) Parenting dysfunction (e.g., harsh, inadequate)
2) Abuse (physical, mental, sexual)
3) Neglect
4) Poverty
5) Bullying
6) Syndromes (autism, fragile X, etc.)
7) Medical conditions
   - ADHD
   - Seizure disorder
   - CNS lesions
   - Medications, e.g., stimulants
8) Learning disabilities
9) Exposure to violence (family, societal)
10) Underlying mental health conditions
    - Anxiety/depression
    - ODD/CD

   PEARL: When the underlying cause is environmental (e.g., parenting dysfunction or bullying), the initial approach should focus on elimination or minimization of the obvious risk factor.

   PEARL: More than one risk factor is usually/often seen in any given patient.

Diagnosis of aggression

Rule: The diagnosis of aggression is no different than our approach to any medical or mental health condition.

1) Thorough history: Family, social, educational, developmental, behavior history, including current family dynamics.
   - How/when/where is aggression precipitated?
   - What worsens it?
   - What improves it?
   - Is it lessening or worsening?
   - What treatments have been tried?
   - What were the results of the treatment?
2) Physical examination
   - Rule out (R/O) chronic illness, neurologic disorder
   - R/O syndrome, physical defects
3) 1:1 Interview with child/adolescent (review again sections in chapter 3 re: interviewing the ADHD child, and chapter 12 re: the mental health interview for Mood Disorders.)
   - Assess mood. R/O anxiety/depression
   - Assess child's insight to the problem
   - Child/adolescent perception of symptoms; what triggers, worsens, improves, etc.
4) Screening tools (e.g., rating scales)
   The following tools are helpful in both screening for underlying causes of aggression or quantitating the degree of symptoms.
   see chapter 1 on Rating Scales for questionnaires, how to score, etc.
   - Modified Overt Aggression Scale
   - Nisonger Child Behavior Rating Form
   - Child Behavior Checklist
   - Patient Health Questionnaire-9 (depression)
   - Screen for Child Anxiety Disorders (SCARED, anxiety)
   - Vanderbilt (ADHD)
5) Other information
   - Review of report cards since kindergarten
   - Observations from teacher, family counselor, 1:1 therapist, school psychologist, etc.
   - Any other reports such as educational, behavioral
   - **PEARL:** If the child/adolescent had speech/language therapy at a younger age, then consider repeating the evaluation by specifically assessing the patient's pragmatic usage of language, as aggression can be a result of inappropriate language interpretation.
6) Laboratory tests (if indicated)
   - Genetic testing (e.g., fragile X)
   - Substance abuse

Treatment of the aggressive child

1) Develop treatment plan with family
   - Discuss details of treatment, goals, monitoring
   - Parent support group
   - Other parent resources are books, organizations, Internet, etc.
2) Eliminate/minimize underlying risk factors or causes such as abuse, neglect, bullying, parenting dysfunction, exposure to violence, etc.
3) If there are academic difficulties test for learning disabilities and remediate (tutor, special education, etc.)
4) Strongly consider referral to a mental health counselor to provide
   - parenting help, e.g., symptom management, *1-2-3 magic* technique;
   - education regarding cause, prevention, monitoring, etc.;
   - 1:1 therapy for child/adolescent;
   - help in coordinating with schools regarding monitoring and symptom management in the classroom.
5) If the patient needs more intensive treatment then try
   - behavior classroom,
   - summer camp/school behavioral programs,
   - medications (see following discussion),
   - potential residential placement (as the last resort).

Medication treatment for an aggressive child/adolescent

1) Treat with maximum dose for any underlying mental health condition; e.g., for ADHD prescribe a stimulant medication prior to the initiation of atypical antipsychotic medication, SSRIs for anxiety/depression, etc.
2) Use of atypical antipsychotic medication to be considered only if both a maximum dose of a specific medication (e.g., stimulant for ADHD) and intensive behavior interventions are not able to control the aggressive symptoms.
3) Obtain baseline laboratory and physical information prior to starting the medication. Baseline data needed prior to the initiation of atypical antipsychotic medication include (see also chapters 13 and 16 regarding treatment with Atypical Antipsychotic medication.)

- height, weight, body mass index;
- Measuring hemoglobin/hematocrit, lipid screen, prolactin, fasting blood sugar levels, thyroid, alanine aminotransferase (ALT) levels.

4) Consider a trial with risperidone (has most research data in pediatrics)
   - Start low, go slow
   - Starting daily dosage
     Children, 0.25 mg
     Adolescents, 0.50 mg
   - May increase every 3–4 days by 0.25–0.5 mg
   - Target dosages (maximum)
     Child, 1.5–2.0 mg/day
     Adolescent, 2–4 mg/day
   - Reach target dose at 2 weeks or so
   - Full efficacy at 4–6 weeks
5) Side effects (can be mild to severe)
   - Weight gain
   - Increase in prolactin levels
   - Increase in blood sugar, triglyceride, and ALT levels
   - See Chapter 16 for more information on atypical antipsychotic medications.
6) Monitor laboratory work, weight, etc. every 3 months
7) If not successful in controlling symptoms, then refer to child psychiatry

REFERENCES

1. Knapp P, et al. Treatment of maladaptive aggression in youth: CERT guidelines I. Engagement, assessment, and management. *Pediatrics* 129:e1562, 2012. Published online 28 May 2012. https://doi.org/10.1542/peds.2010-1360.
2. Rosato N, et al. Treatment of maladaptive aggression in youth: CERT guidelines II. Treatments and ongoing management. *Pediatrics* 129:e1577, 2012. Published online 28 May 2012. https://doi.org/10.1542/peds.2010-1361.

RESOURCE

"The T-MAY Toolkit re: management of aggressive behaviors is a 38 page document that can be downloaded free from the following website: www.thereachinstitute.org/guidelines-for-adolescent-depression-primary-care/2-uncategorized/125-treatment-maladaptive-aggression-youth"

T-MAY RECOMMENDATIONS FOR AGGRESSION

T-MAY RECOMMENDATIONS

ASSESSMENT + DIAGNOSIS

- ☐ Engage patients and parents (emphasize need for their on-going participation)
- ☐ Conduct a thorough initial evaluation and diagnostic work-up before initiating treatment
- ☐ Define target symptoms and behaviors in partnership with parents and child
- ☐ Assess target symptoms, treatment effects and outcomes with standardized measures

INITIAL TREATMENT + MANAGEMENT PLANNING

- ☐ Conduct a risk assessment and if needed, consider referral to mental health specialist or ER
- ☐ Partner with family in developing an acceptable treatment plan
- ☐ Provide psychoeducation and help families form realistic expectations about treatment
- ☐ Help the family to establish community and social supports

PSYCHOSOCIAL INTERVENTIONS

- ☐ Provide or assist the family in obtaining evidence-based parent and child skills training
- ☐ Identify, assess and address the child's social, educational and family needs, and set objectives and outcomes with the family
- ☐ Engage child and family in maintaining consistent psychological/behavioral strategies

MEDICATION TREATMENTS

- ☐ Select initial medication treatment to target the underlying disorder(s); follow guidelines for primary disorder (when available)
- ☐ If severe aggression persists following adequate trials of appropriate psychosocial and medication treatments for underlying disorder, add an AP, try a different AP, or augment with a mood stabilizer (MS)
- ☐ Avoid using more than two psychotropic medications simultaneously
- ☐ Use the recommended titration schedule and deliver an adequate medication trial before adjusting medication

SIDE-EFFECT MANAGEMENT

- ☐ Assess side-effects, and do clinically-relevant metabolic studies and laboratory tests based on established guidelines and schedule
- ☐ Provide accessible information to children and parents about identifying and managing side-effects
- ☐ Use evidence-based strategies to prevent or reduce side-effects
- ☐ Collaborate with medical, educational and/or mental health specialists if needed

MEDICATION MAINTENANCE + DISCONTINUATION

- ☐ If response is favorable, continue treatment for six months.
- ☐ Taper or discontinue medications in patients who show a remission in aggressive symptoms ≥ 6 months

Note: The order of these recommendations may be tailored to each patient's specific condition and needs.

4

WHAT IS DISRUPTIVE MOOD DYSREGULATION DISORDER?

Disruptive mood dysregulation disorder (DMDD) is a new diagnostic category to apply to the child who has chronic irritability and behavioral outbursts.

It's incidence is 2%–5%.

Characteristics:

1) Chronic irritability, or angry mood, most of the days.
2) Verbal and/or physical outbursts, sometimes aggressive in nature, occurring several times weekly, in multiple settings, for a year or more.
3) Outbursts would not be considered appropriate for the child's age.
4) Mostly seen in males, mostly prior to 10 years of age.
5) More likely to transition into anxiety/mood disorder than bipolar disorder.
6) Frequently coexistent with ADHD and/or anxiety and mood disorders.
7) DMDD is distinguished from ODD by the relative absence of chronic mood symptoms in ODD, so DMDD and ODD are not coexistent disorders.

Differential diagnosis: Borderline personality disorder, ODD, ADHD, depression/anxiety, autism.

Treatment: Depends on the symptoms and related coexistent conditions.

PEARL: Would recommend psychiatric help with this complicated problem. Usual course would be to surface early with behavior problems and aggressive behavior, so ODD would be an early consideration, but the chronic mood symptoms (irritability, anger) would R/O ODD and suggest DMDD.

PEARL: If you see an adolescent with an altered mental state, and a negative result in drug screening, it may suggest synthetic cannabinoid use (which would not show up when screening).

PEARL: Here's a potential quick screen.

Researchers at the National Institutes of Health (in April 2016) developed a one-question screen that they used for a large group of 12- to 17-year-old adolescents: "Did you have at least one drink on three or more days last year?"

Results: Those who said "Yes" were subsequently shown to have an alcohol use disorder, with 91% sensitivity and 93% specificity.

CHAPTER 15

Medications for ADHD

CURRENT FDA-APPROVED MEDICATIONS FOR ADHD

Medications	Available Forms (mg)	Initial Dose (mg)	Peak Dose (h)	Duration (h)	Comments
Medications for ADHD: Amphetamines and Nonstimulants (Brand Names are Listed. Some Have Generic Forms.) Harlan R. Gephart, MD					
AMPHETAMINES (BRAND NAMES)					
Short Acting					
Adderall	5, 7.5, 10, 12.5, 15, 20, 30	5	3	4–6	Highly abused
Dextrostat (dextroamphetamine)	5, 10	5	3	4–6	Highly abused
ProCenta	5 mg/5 mL	5	2–4	4–6	May cause Raynaud phenomenon
Long Acting					
Vyvanse	20, 30, 40, 50, 60, 70	20	3.5–4.5	8–12	Capsule can be opened and sprinkled or dissolved in liquid. CANNOT BE ABUSED BY SNORTING.
Adderall XR	5, 10, 15, 20, 30	5	3–5	8–12	Highly abused
Dexedrine spansule	5, 10, 15	5	3–4	6–10	Highly abused
[a]Adzenys XR-ODT	3.1, 6.3, 9.4, 12.5, 15.7, 18.8	3.1 or 6.3	5	10–11	ALLOW PILL TO FIRST DISSOLVE ON TONGUE
[a]Dyanavel XR (suspension)	2.5 mg/mL	2.5–5.0	1	13	Maximum dose, 20.0 mg
NONSTIMULANTS					
α-Agonists/Long Acting					
Intuniv (guanfacine)	1, 2, 3, 4	1		8–12	Maximum dose for ages 6–12 years, 4 mg ages 13–17 years, 7 mg
Kapvay (clonidine)	0.1	0.1 (greater doses should be split bid)		8–12	If discontinued need to taper 0.1 mg every 3–7 days. Maximum dose, 0.4 mg

Continued

Medications for ADHD: Amphetamines and Nonstimulants (Brand Names are Listed. Some Have Generic Forms.) Harlan R. Gephart, MD—cont'd

Medications	Available Forms (mg)	Initial Dose (mg)	Peak Dose (h)	Duration (h)	Comments
Antidepressant					
Strattera (atomoxetine)	10, 18, 25, 40, 60, 80, 100	0.5 mg/kg per day. In 2 weeks, 1.2 mg/kg per day. Do not exceed 1.4 mg/kg per day.	Target 1.2 mg/kg per day Do not exceed 1.4 mg/kg per day	18–24	See some effect at 1–2 weeks, peak at 2–4 weeks BOX WARNING!

[a] New.

Medications for ADHD: Methylphenidates (Brand Names are Listed. Some Have Generic Forms.) Harlan R. Gephart, MD

Brand Name	Available Forms (mg)	Initial Dose (mg)	Peak Dose (h)	Duration (h)	Comments
SHORT ACTING					
Ritalin	5, 10, 20	5.0	2–3	4	
Focalin	2.5, 5, 10	2.5	2–3	4–5	Twice as strong as other methylphenidates
Methylin	5, 10, 20	5.0	2–3	4–6	
Methylin chewable	2.5, 5, 10	2.5	2–3	4–6	
Methylin solution	5 mg/5 mL and 10 mg/5 mL	5	2–4	4	
LONG ACTING (8–12 H)					
Concerta	18, 27, 36, 54	18	6–8	8–12	
Focalin XR	5, 10, 15, 20	5	3–4	8–12	Twice as strong as other methylphenidates
Ritalin LA	10, 20, 30, 40	10	3–5	4–8	
Metadate CD	10, 20, 30, 40, 50, 60	10	3–5	4–8	
Ritalin SR	20	20	3–4	6–8	Old medication; unreliable
Methylin ER	10, 20	10	3–5	4–8	
[a]Quillivant XR (liquid)	25 mg/5 mL	1–2 mL	45 min	8–12	
[a]QuilliChew ER (chewable)	20, 30, 40	20	45 min	8	
[a]Aptensio XR	10, 15, 20, 30, 40, 50, 60	10	Effects seen at 1 h	12	Capsules may be opened and sprinkled
Daytrana patch	10, 15, 20, 30	10	2	12 h plus 3 h after patch removed	May cause skin rash

[a] New.

Addendum: Four pharmaceutical companies have recently received FDA approval to market generic atomoxetine (Strattera). They are Apotex, Teva Pharmaceutical Industries, Aurobindo Pharma, and Glenmark Pharma.

RISK OF MEDICATION ABUSE/DIVERSION

1) Self-medication: About 5% of college students (various sources) illicitly used stimulants in the past year (most commonly, Adderall).

   - To study better for tests
   - Less likely to get "high"

2) Diversion (Wilens, *JAACAP* 2006)
   - About 22% of adolescents with ADHD misused their prescribed medications
   - About 11% sold their medications
   - One-third of adolescents have "tried medications"

Risks of giving or selling one's medications should be discussed prior to initiation of treatment. For example, perhaps another adolescent has an undiagnosed heart condition, for whom stimulant medications might be life-threatening.

Stress that some medicines need to be tapered, e.g., selective serotonin reuptake inhibitors.

ISSUES TO BE ADDRESSED PRIOR TO ADMINISTRATION OF MEDICATIONS

1) Self-image: Adolescent is being treated for a medical condition, not being "drugged" by the clinician.
2) Friends may say, "I don't like you on medications" (because of a decrease in inappropriate behaviors, such as blurting out in class).
3) Side effects: Potential, acceptable/not acceptable.
4) "Loss of creativity" and "zombie feeling": Almost always due to too large a dose.
5) Risk to others if medications diverted, for example, potential unknown cardiac risk.
6) Necessity for compliance, not sporadic usage or dosage variation.
7) Risks of inappropriate usage, for example, snorting vs. ingesting.
8) Risks if other substances are used (e.g., pot, alcohol) when taking medications.
9) Need for frequent monitoring (appointments, school reports, etc.).
10) The good news! Most children/adolescents (~80%–90% informal data from our large clinic) who take ADHD medications will not need them as adults, hopefully due to having an interesting and motivating job and the burden of school being lifted after high school or college (many do not find medications necessary after 2–3 years of college). ADHD symptoms actually do lessen with age for many patients, and the adolescent/adult also learns coping skills that also minimize symptoms.

PEARL: Remember, however, that even though the ADHD symptoms are lessened, or maybe not recognizable enough for an ADHD diagnosis, the adolescent/adult might well be left with a comorbid condition, such as anxiety or depression, and need help with that.

RECENT MEDICATIONS APPROVED BY THE FDA FOR ADHD TREATMENT

1) **Adzenys XR-ODT** (Neos Therapeutics)
   An amphetamine
   For ages 6 years and over
   Has both immediate and long-acting effects
   Orally disintegrates and can be taken without water
2) **Quillivant XR** (Pfizer Ltd.)
   A long-acting liquid methylphenidate
   For ages 6 years and over
3) **QuilliChew ER** (Pfizer Ltd.)
   A long-acting chewable methylphenidate
   For ages 6 years and over
4) **Dyanavel XR** (Tris Pharma)
   A long-acting amphetamine suspension
   For ages 6 years and over
5) **Mydayis** (Shire Plc.)
   Long-acting mixed amphetamine salts
   For ages 13 years and over, including adults
   Onset, 2–4 h; lasts up to 16 h
   Available from late fall 2017
6) **Cotempla XR-ODT** (Neos Therapeutics)
   A methylphenidate extended-release oral medicine; disintegrating
   For ages 6–17 years
   Available doses: 17.3, 25.9, 34.6, and 51.8 mg
   Onset, 1 h; duration, 12 h
   Available from fall 2017
7) **New generic Concerta** (Helio.com)
   Doses: 18, 27, 36, and 54 mg

PEARL: One must always be cautious when prescribing oral liquid medications, as there is a body of evidence that the doses given to the child vary widely ("not every teaspoon is 5 mL!"), unless one provides a measured spoon or dropper.

PEARL: August 2016 *Journal of the American Academy of Child and Adolescent Psychiatry.*

Three studies suggest combinations of medications, e.g., stimulants and α-agonists (e.g., Intuniv, Kapvay), may give greater clinical improvement than when used alone.

We noted this result in our clinic years ago, with both α-agonists and atomoxetine (see the section "What to do when your favorite ADHD medication doesn't work in the ADHD treatment chapter 4"). This research should help us get two medications simultaneously covered by healthcare insurers, which has been somewhat of a struggle to date.

However, our goal should always be to maximize a response to one medication and avoid multiple medications if at all possible.

PEARL: Dr. William Brinkman presented data from a National Institute of Mental Health study (394 kids) at the Pediatric Academic Societies in May 2016, regarding teenagers who stop their ADHD medication on their own. He noted that

- almost all teens stop medications at some point,
- only ~28% restart them,
- the reasons given were
  - "Felt I could do OK without it."
  - "Wanted to see if I could do without it."
  - "Tired of taking it."
  - "Side effects."
  - "Parents stopped it."

We need to be aware of these concerns, perhaps even participate in (and supervise) a controlled trial on and off medications.

Most teenagers with ADHD do not do well if they stop their medications, in our experience and based on at least some limited research data. The experience from our large clinic was that most adolescents who are on ADHD medications need to continue them (perhaps in decreasing doses) through high school and into college for 1−2 years, before considering a trial off of them.

PEARL: It was mentioned earlier that generic medications are sometimes not as effective as the brand name medications, and careful observation is needed when going from brand name to generic medications. On October 18, 2016, FDA removed two generic medications (generic forms of Concerta, a long-acting methylphenidate) from its approved list, one manufactured by Mallinckrodt and the other by UCB/Kremers Urban, formerly Kudco.

The reasons for removal are

a) failed to demonstrate bioequivalence to the brand name medication,

b) may not have the same therapeutic benefits as the brand name medication.

In August 2018 the FDA approved a new ADHD methylphenidate medication (Brand name Jornay PM), manufactured by Ironshore Pharmaceuticals, for evening usage, at an initial dose of 20 mg given between 6:30 PM and 9:00 PM to children 6 years and older, to enable control of ADHD in the early AM the following day. It should be on the market early 2019.

CHAPTER 16

Medications for Other Non-ADHD Mental Health Conditions in Children and Adolescents: Antidepressants and Atypical Antipsychotics

TREATING ADHD SYMPTOMS IN OTHER NON-ADHD CONDITIONS

1) There are several medical conditions, syndromes, etc., where core signs and symptoms of ADHD traits can be present as part of the condition/syndrome (hyperactivity, inattention, impulsivity) (not a complete list):

- Fetal alcohol syndrome (ADHD traits almost universal in the fully expressed syndrome)
- Fragile X syndrome
- William's syndrome
- Turner's syndrome
- Traumatic brain injury
- Near drowning
- Neonatal hypoxia/cerebral palsy
- Autistic spectrum

2) Many of these children are severely impacted by inattention and overactivity.
3) Stimulant medications can sometimes be helpful in reducing these symptoms.
4) The success rate is much less, however, than in typical ADHD patients. Side effects are more likely to occur and at lower doses.
5) Use the same approach as mentioned in treating preschool ADHD children.
   - Start low (small doses of short-acting methylphenidate, for example, 2.5 mg bid).
   - Go slow. Monitor carefully for undesirable side effects (sleep, appetite, agitation, etc.).
   - If tolerated, then often possible to switch to a long-acting preparation.

6) If improvement in symptoms is noted (for example, lessened hyperactivity, better focus), you will have helped the child, and parents and teachers will be gratified.

PEARL: NAMI (National Association for Mental Illness) reported in April 2016 that 70% of kids in the juvenile justice system have a mental health condition and only 50% of kids with mental health issues received treatment in the prior year. We can and should do better!

BOX WARNING

Source: ParentsMedGuide.org.

Joint Statement of APA and AACAP (edited)

In any given year, about 16% of high school students think about suicide and about 3%–8% show suicidal behaviors. Most of them, however, do not commit suicide. If untreated, the risk of depressed adolescents committing suicide is increased. The current rate of adolescent suicide in the United States is 1 in 13,000–14,000 (about 4600 children/adolescents/young adults in the 10- to 24-year-old range).

From 1992 to 2001, with the large increase in antidepressant medicine usage in depressed adolescents, there was a marked decrease (about 25%) in the rate of suicides in adolescents. This was the first decline in the suicide rate in many years.

In 2004, the FDA reviewed many clinical trial reports, almost all from pharmaceutical companies, which suggested that there was an increase in suicidal ideation (thoughts or behaviors) in the adolescent participants in these drug trials, although there was no associated increase in actual suicide occurrences.

The rate of suicidal ideation was about 4% (more recent study suggests a rate of 3%) compared with a baseline rate of 2% suicidal ideation in children/adolescents not taking medication although having the same diagnosis.

The studies that were reviewed by FDA were in some ways flawed, e.g., by small sample size, selection bias, lack of uniformity, and of short duration. Again, it is important to emphasize that in the 4400 or so children and adolescents (in the studies) who were given antidepressant medication for major depression, anxiety, or obsessive compulsive disorder, there were no suicides that were successful, although there were a few unsuccessful attempts.

In 2004, the FDA imposed a Box Warning (initially called Black Box Warning) on all antidepressant medication given to children and adolescents, basically stating that such medications are "associated with an increased risk of suicidal thinking and/or behavior in a small proportion of children and adolescents, especially during the early phases of treatment."

This warning applied not only to the SSRI antidepressants but also included the TCAs (tricyclic antidepressants, e.g., desipramine, etc.) as well as the antidepressant atomoxetine, which is helpful for ADHD patients.

In 2007, the warning was extended to young adults aged 18–24 years.

Interestingly, following the release of the Box Warning, there was a significant decline in the prescription rates of antidepressant medication for children and youth, presumably due to physician and parent concerns. At the same time, from 2003 to 2004, there was noted an increase in suicide rate among youth, the first such increase in many years. Whether these two observable facts are causally related cannot be verified, although many experts presume they are.

What is the primary care clinician's role in this whole discussion? First and foremost, it is important to discuss with adolescents and patients the conclusions of the FDA and what the Box Warning means. Again, emphasize that no actual suicides occurred in any of the research groups. It is indeed possible, however, that temporarily a small percentile of medicated patients (1%–2%) have an increase in suicidal ideation just after the initiation of medication,

compared with patients with similar diagnoses but are nonmedicated.

Also, it is crucial to discuss the serious nature of major depression in children and youth, *and the risk of suicide if left untreated.*

Lastly, and most importantly, the above discussion should focus on the treatment of major depression in children and youth, which should involve, along with medication:
1) Counseling: Cognitive behavior therapy (CBT) or interpersonal.
2) Suicidal precautions regarding guns, knives, medications/drugs.
3) Close monitoring by a healthcare provider.

In summary, I want to quote Dr. Cathryn Galanter, Visiting Associate Professor of Psychiatry, SUNY Downstate/Kings County Hospital Center and member of the REACH faculty, who recently stated the following:
- Antidepressants treat depression.
- Suicide is a risk with depression.
- Suicide is a rare event.
- No suicides occurred in children and teens in the research studies.
- Suicidal ideation decreases with antidepressant treatment, especially when CBT is part of the treatment. (Source: TADS Study: "Treatment for Adolescent Depression Study," in the section on Clinical Studies that the Clinician Should Read.)
- It is important to monitor and educate.
- The Box Warning is relevant for kids, teens, and young adults.

PRACTICE PARAMETERS FOR THE USE OF ATYPICAL ANTIPSYCHOTIC MEDICATIONS IN CHILDREN AND ADOLESCENTS

Case Vignette: Jared is a 7-year-old first-grade child, whose parents came to see you because of his aggressive behavior. He had been diagnosed with ADHD, combined type, at the age of 5 years while attending Kindergarten. Symptoms included hyperactivity, impulsivity, and inattentiveness. He refused to sit still in "circle time" but instead wandered around the room making noise and disrupting the class. He was treated with ADHD medications, to maximum doses, but eventually was asked to leave the school. Parents were told he "wasn't ready for school."

He was kept at home for another year, and parents received 1:1 counseling in behavior therapy from a child psychologist, which along with his medication seemed to control his behavior somewhat. He was then enrolled in first grade. It was noted that Jared continued to relate poorly to other children, had stereotypic behaviors such as "rocking," and became increasingly aggressive, both toward his peers as well as the teacher and her aide. This was despite his being in a small behavioral classroom of eight students. Parents say his aggressiveness is manifested by kicking and biting his classmates as well as his teachers, and even occasionally his parents.

Your advice was to seek consultation with a child psychiatrist, who made an additional diagnosis of autistic spectrum disorder, and a recommendation of adding an atypical antipsychotic medication to his current ADHD medications.

Author Preface

As mentioned in chapter 13 on Psychosis and Bipolar Disorder, it is not the intention of this handbook to make primary care clinicians into "mini child psychiatrists." Obviously, children and adolescents with diagnoses such as schizophrenia and bipolar disorder should be diagnosed and followed by our colleagues in psychiatry.

However, having said that, these patients will come from our own practice pool, and we will be responsible for their overall health and welfare. It behooves us, therefore, to not only be able to recognize the signs and symptoms of these uncommon conditions but also to know how they are treated, particularly the medications, dosages, etc.

And, most importantly, monitor for the possible significant side effects that may occur. In that sense, we in primary care should see ourselves in partnership with our colleagues in psychiatry in providing the optimal therapeutic environment for our joint patient. This will take some effort on our part, not only in communicating with our colleagues but also in learning about these uncommon but complex conditions and their treatment. One condition where atypical antipsychotic medication might not only be helpful but indicated is illustrated by the case vignette described in the previous section, the aggressive 7 year-old child whose diagnoses are both ADHD and Autistic Spectrum Disorder.

So, with that preface, let us talk about the use of atypical antipsychotic medication.

Reference: American Academy of Child and Adolescent Psychiatry, August 2011 Guidelines for Use of Atypical Antipsychotic Medications.

A. Medications that are FDA approved for use in children and adolescents (and specific indications)
 1) Risperidone, aripiprazole: Autistic disorder (irritability, aggressiveness)
 2) Risperidone, aripiprazole, olanzapine, quetiapine: Adolescents with schizophrenia, bipolar disorder.
B. Current "off-label" use: Other conditions in pediatric patients, e.g., ADHD with aggression, disruptive behavior disorders, Tourette syndrome, OCD, depression, etc. (more used for targeting aggressive symptoms than psychosis!).
C. Facts
 1) Atypical antipsychotics each have different safety profiles, as well as efficacy and tolerability, in individual patients.
 2) Risperidone has the most research about its use in children and adolescents; for example, severe behavior problems in autistic children. It has also shown to be helpful in children with disruptive behavior disorders, behavior disorders in borderline or low IQ, and impulsive aggression in conduct disorder.
 3) Risperidone is currently recommended in the Texas ADHD algorithm for children with ADHD and aggression, who are not controlled by stimulant medication and behavior therapy.
 4) Overall: Best evidence for use of atypical antipsychotics is in children and adolescents with schizophrenia and bipolar disorder, as well as in autism with disruptive behavior disorder, and less robust evidence regarding efficacy in other disruptive behavior disorders.
 5) There is paucity of data in all the atypical antipsychotics regarding long-term efficacy and safety.

PEARL: Remember the three FDA approved uses of atypical antipsychotics in children and adolescents: (1) Autism with irritability and disruptive behavior; (2) Schizophrenia; (3) Juvenile bipolar disorder. All other uses are off-label. Patients for consideration of these meds off-label should be on a case by case basis, presumably in most cases with consultation from a child/adolescent psychiatrist. This is due to the severe nature of some of the side effects of these meds (see below), as well as lack of information about their effect on the developing brain.
(It has been heartening in recent years to see a decline in the prescription of these medications for off-label considerations.)

D. Side effects and safety

Important: There are several significant side effects associated with the usage of atypical antipsychotic medication, which are listed below. *some are irreversible*! Prior to usage, it is critical that the clinician carefully considers the risk versus the potential benefit (for each patient). Prepubertal children are more vulnerable!

1) **Weight gain, diabetes, hyperlipidemia.** All atypical antipsychotic medications have a Box Warning regarding the risk of patients developing diabetes, through weight gain and insulin resistance.

2) **Cardiovascular.** Potential side effects include prolonged QTc interval, orthostatic hypotension, tachycardia, and pericarditis, some of which might be worsened by excessive weight gain.

3) **Agranulocytosis and neutropenia.**

4) **Hepatic dysfunction**: This appears to be relatively uncommon, possibly related to rapid weight gain, suggesting that in that scenario liver function should be monitored.

5) **Prolactin elevation.** More common with risperidone. Possible symptoms include gynecomastia, amenorrhea, etc., but long-term effect on growth and puberty is not known.

6) **Seizures.** EEG changes can be noted, but risk for seizures seems minimal.

7) **Extrapyramidal symptoms, Tardive dyskinesia, and withdrawal dyskinesias.** Movement disorders which, although uncommon, can be permanent and, therefore, a source of considerable patient consternation.

8) **Neuroleptic malignant syndrome.** Very rare, with symptoms of autonomic instability, elevated temperature, rigidity, elevated creatine phosphokinase, and potentially fatal.

9) **Cataracts.** Potential complication in adults, not so far in youth.

E. Screening and assessment recommendations

1) The general guidelines that pertain to the prescription of psychotropic medications should be followed, including a thorough discussion of potential risks and benefits with both the adolescent and parent/caretakers.

2) When prescribing an atypical antipsychotic medication, clinician should follow most recent evidence in scientific literature.

3) Prior to initiation of treatment, clinician should obtain thorough patient and family history of diabetes, hyperlipidemia, seizures, and cardiac abnormalities.

4) Dosing should follow the "start low and go slow" approach and seek to find the lowest effective dose.

5) Target dose should be supported by current medical literature and will vary depending on the condition being treated.

6) If side effects occur, a trial at a lower dose should be considered; however, certain side effects may preclude further treatment with the specific atypical antipsychotic.

7) The use of multiple psychotropic medications in refractory patients may, at times, be necessary but has not been studied rigorously, and clinicians should proceed with caution.

8) The simultaneous use of multiple atypical antipsychotics has not been studied rigorously and generally should be avoided.

9) After the failure of one atypical antipsychotic, the selection of an alternative medication may include consideration of another atypical antipsychotic and/or a medication from a different class of drugs.

10) The acute and long-term safety of these medications in children and adolescents has not been fully evaluated and, therefore, careful and frequent monitoring of side effects should be performed.

11) BMI should be obtained at baseline and monitored at regular intervals throughout treatment with an atypical antipsychotic.

12) Careful attention should be given to the increased risk of developing diabetes with the use of an atypical antipsychotic, and blood glucose levels and other parameters should be obtained at baseline and monitored at regular intervals.

13) In those patients with significant weight changes and/or a family history indicating high risk, lipid profiles should be obtained at baseline and monitored at regular intervals.

14) Measurements of movement disorders using structured measures, such as the Abnormal Involuntary Movement Scale, should be done at baseline and at regular intervals during treatment and during tapering of the atypical antipsychotic medication.

15) Due to limited data surrounding the impact of atypical antipsychotics on the cardiovascular system, regular monitoring of heart rate, blood pressure, and EKG changes should be performed.

16) Although there is a relationship between atypical antipsychotic use and elevations of prolactin, the current state of evidence does not support the need for routine monitoring of prolactin levels in asymptomatic youths.

17) Due to drug-specific risks, additional monitoring should be considered for specific atypical antipsychotic medications.

18) The limited long-term safety and efficacy data warrant careful consideration, before the initiation of medication, of the planned duration of the medication trial.

19) Abrupt discontinuation of a medication is not recommended!

Reprinted with permission of the American Academy of Child and Adolescent Psychiatry. (AACAP). The term "Practice Parameters" has recently been changed by the AACAP to "Clinical practice Guidelines." The Practice Parameter quoted above will be revised in 2017, due to new research and medical literature, to a new "Clinical Practice Guideline for the use of Atypical Antipsychotic Medication" and will be available on the AACAP website under "Resources for Primary Care."

Disclaimer:

The information on the cards (antipsychotic and mood stabilizer medications) contains general guidelines and do not mean to be clinical recommendations for individual patients.

Usual Antipsychotic and Mood Stabilizer Medication Dosing and Titration Levels (Reprinted With the Permission of the Resource for Advancing Children's Health (REACH) Institute, Patient-Centered Mental Health in Primary Care (PPP) Program Copyright.)

USUAL MEDICATION DOSING AND TITRATION INTERVALS OF ANTIPSYCHOTICS (APs) *

ANTIPSYCHOTIC	DOSE RANGE (mg)	DOSE STRENGTH (mg)	MEDICATION FORMULATIONS (available for use)	STARTING DOSE (mg)	HALF LIFE (hrs)	TIME TO PEAK (hrs)	TITRATION INTERVALS (days)	PRINCIPAL LIVER ENZYME	LIVER ENZYME INDUCER	LIVER ENZYME INHIBITOR
SECOND GENERATION ANTIPSYCHOTICS (SGA)										
ARIPIPRAZOLE (ARI)	Child: 2.5 - 15 Adol: 5 to 15	2, 5, 10, 15, 20, 30 tbl; 10, 15 diss, liquid 1 (30 mg = 25 mL)	po, im short, diss., liquid	2 to 5 ---- Chlorpromazine Dose ≈ 7.5mg	50 to 72	3 to 5	when starting at 2mg, may increase dose every 3rd day; after steady state, increase dose every 7-14 days	2D6 > 3A4	3A4	2D6 3A4
CLOZAPINE (CLO)	Child: 150 - 300 Adol: 200 - 600	25; 100	po	12.5 ---- Chlorpromazine Dose ≈ 50 mg	12	1 to 4	25 mg daily or, every other day	1A2>2C19 2C19>3A4 3A4 > 2C9 2C9 > 2D6	1A2 2C19 3A4	1A2 2C19 3A4 2C9
OLANZAPINE (OLA)	N/A	.5, 5, 7.5, 10, 15, 20 tb 5, 10, 15, 20 diss; 10im	po, im short, diss.	5 to 10 Chlorpromazine Dose ≈ 5 mg	30	6	increase at intervals > 5 days	1A2 2D6 3A4	1A2 2D6 3A4	1A2 2D6 3A4
PALIPERIDONE (PAL)	3 to 12	3, 6, 9	po, ER	3 Chlorpromazine Dose ≈ 3 mg	21 to 30	24	increase at intervals > 5 days	<10% Hepatic Clearance	N/A	N/A
QUETIAPINE (QUE)	150 to 750	25, 100, 200	po, XR	50-100 IR 200-300 XR Chlorpromazine Dose ≈ 75 mg	6 to 7	2	100 mg per day	3A4	3A4	3A4
RISPERIDONE (RIS)	Child: 1.5 - 2 Adol: 2 to 4	0.5, 1, 2, 3, 4 tablets; 0.5, 1, 2 diss; liquid 1mg/mL 30ml bottl	po, im long, diss., liquid	0.5 to 1 ---- Chlorpromazine Dose ≈ 2 mg	3	1 to 2	increase at intervals of 0.5-1 per day or > 5 days	2D6 > 3A4	2D6 3A4	2D6 3A4
ZIPRASIDONE (ZIP)	80 to 160	20, 40, 60, 80 tablets	po im short	20 to 40 Chlorpromazine Dose ≈ 60 mg	7	5	increase at 20- 40 per day	Aldehyde Oxidase > 3A4	3A4	3A4

Modified from: Correll 2008 (Correll CU). Antipsychotics and Adjunctive Medications. In: Textbook of a Child and Adolescent Psychiatry. M Dulcan (ed.), American Psychiatric Publishing, Inc. New York.

Modified from: 2004 .TRAAY - A Pocket Reference Guide. New York State Office of Mental Health, Research Foundation for Mental Hygiene, Inc. and the Trustees of Columbia University.

TYPICAL MEDICATION DOSING AND TITRATION INTERVALS OF ANTIPSYCHOTICS *

ANTIPSYCHOTIC	DOSE RANGE (mg)	DOSE STRENGTH (mg)	MEDICATION FORMULATIONS (available for use)	STARTING DOSE (mg)	HALF LIFE (hrs)	TIME TO PEAK (hrs)	TITRATION INTERVALS (days)	PRINCIPAL LIVER ENZYME	LIVER ENZYME INDUCER	LIVER ENZYME INHIBITOR
FIRST GENERATION ANTIPSYCHOTICS (FGA)										
HALOPERIDOL (HAL)	1 to 6	0.5, 1, 2, 5, 10, 20 tablets, 2; 10 mg/mL liquid, 5 im	po, im short, im long	0.25-1 / Chlorpromazine Dose ≈ 2 mg	3 - 6 po / 10-20 im	2-6 po / .05 im	increase dose by 0.5 kg intervals of 5-7 days	3A4	3A4	3A4
MOLINDONE (MOL)	20 to 140	5, 10, 25, 50	po	0.5-1 mg/kg/d divided in 3-4 doses Chlorpromazine Dose ≈ 10 mg	1.5	1.5	N/A	2D6	2D6	2D6
PERPHENAZINE (PER)	8 to 32	2, 4, 8, 16	po	TBD; no data available Chlorpromazine Dose ≈ 10 mg	8 to 12	1 to 3	TBD; no data available	2D6	2D6	2D6

Modified from: Correll 2008 (Correll CU). Antipsychotics + Adjunctive Medications. Textbook of a Child + Adolescent Psychiatry. M Dulcan (ed.), American Psychiatric Publishing, Inc. New York.

USUAL MEDICATION DOSING AND TITRATION INTERVALS OF MOOD STABILIZERS *

MOOD STABILIZER	DOSE RANGE (mg)	DOSE STRENGTH (mg)	MEDICATION FORMULATIONS (available for use)	STARTING DOSE (mg)	HALF LIFE (hrs)	TIME TO PEAK (hrs)	TITRATION INTERVALS (days)	PRINCIPAL LIVER ENZYME	LIVER ENZYME INDUCER	LIVER ENZYME INHIBITOR
CARBAMAZEPINE	100 - 800	100, 200, 100 mg/5mL	po	100 mg B.I.D. (tbl), 1/2 tsp QID (susp) for 6-12 years	Initial 25 - 65 Later 12 to 17	4 to 5	Add < 100 mg/day at weekly intervals, t.i.d or q.i.d. (tbl) til optimal reponse	3A4>2D6 2D6.1A2 Auto-Inducer	3A4 2D6 1A2	3A4 2D6 1A2
CARBAMAZEPINE ER	100 - 800	100, 200, 400	po	100 mg for 6-12 years B.I.D. or T.I.D.	Initial 25 - 65 Later 12 to 17	3 to 12	Add 100 mg/day at weekly intervals b.i.d until optimal response	3A4>2D6 2D6.1A2 Auto-Inducer	3A4 2D6 1A2	3A4 2D6 1A2
DIVALPROEX	500 - 2000	125, 250, 500	po	10 - 15 mg/kg/d B.I.D. or T.I.D.	9 to 16	3 to 4	Add 5-10 mg/kg day q 7 days; give with food. Increase rapidly to lowest effective dose	CYP450 C29 (weak inhibitor)	Rifampin Seco-barbital	# please see footnote
DIVALPROEX ER	500 - 2000	250, 500	po	10-15 mg/kg/day po	9 to 16	7 to 14	Increase dose by 5 - 10 mg/kg/wk until optimal response; clinical response is at plasma levels of 85-125 µg/mL	CYP450 C29 (weak inhibitor)	Rifampin Seco-barbital	# please see footnote
LAMOTRIGINE	50 - 200	25, 100, 150, 200	po	only 25mg < 16 yo, or on DVP	24 - 34	1.4 - 4.8	Keep starting dose stable for 2 wks, increase by 12.5 - 25 mg; but if < 16 yo, or on DVP, increase by 12.5 mg	Glucu-ronidation	N/A	N/A
LITHIUM	600 - 1800	8mEq/5mL	po	15 - 20 mg/kg/d B.I.D or T.I.D.	20 - 24	1 to 3	Dose wkly based on plasma Li+ levels	Renal Elimination Only	Renal Elimination Only	Renal Elimination Only
LITHIUM CR	1800 mg/d, serum level 1-1.5mEq/L adults	300, 450	po	150 - 300 mg B.I.D.	24	4	Dose according to need	Renal Elimination Only	Renal Elimination Only	Renal Elimination Only

Modified from: Correll and Schenck. Correll CU and Schenck EM. Assessing and Treating Pediatric Bipolar Disorder. Oxford American Psychiatry Library. In preparation.

CHAPTER 17

Office Practice Recommendations for Primary Care Management of Mental Health Issues in Children and Adolescents

USING ONLINE ASSESSMENT TOOLS AND PORTAL

Currently there are online assessment tools commercially available for office use, e.g., to code, collate, summarize, data gathered in clinic settings.

What are the benefits?

1. Eliminate excessive paperwork
2. Streamline assessment procedures
3. Accumulate and maintain databases
4. Improve communication between patients and providers
   Examples of documents saved: Developmental screens, ADHD rating scales, assessing for coexisting problems (learning disorder, anxiety, depression, substance abuse)
5. Quantifying negative behavior, e.g., aggression

The best known system is the Child Health & Development Interactive System (CHADIS). Currently utilized by about 7000 providers, at a cost about $1000 per provider per year.

Parents fill out appropriate screening tools of development, behavior, which are scored and utilized by the provider as needed for assessment of parent concerns or other identified problems. CHADIS also provides treatment resources for the clinician when concerns are diagnosed or identified. All information is easily adaptable to the electronic health record and becomes part of the child's medical record.

A more specific online portal is mehealth for ADHD (Optimal Medicine, Marlborough, Boston, MA), which screens only for ADHD and its associated issues. Again all information from the parents is entered online and eventually becomes part of the patient electronic medical record. The American Academy of Pediatrics (AAP) has initiated an ADHD project using the mehealth system to assess if and/or how it can improve ADHD care.

ADDED BENEFITS: Both mehealth and CHADIS are recognized by the American Board of Pediatrics to fulfill Maintenance of Certification Part 4 credits.

Also, many of the screening tools can be reimbursed so that the fee for the involvement in the online portal system is retrievable (e.g., rating scales are usually reimbursed, such as Vanderbilt, Screen for Child Anxiety Disorders [SCARED], Patient Health Questionnaire (PHQ)-9, but questionnaires that are extensions of the medical history are usually not reimbursed.).

Concerns:

1. Parent inconsistency with completing the forms, e.g., follow-up ADHD rating scales.
2. Reliance on rating scales for diagnosis, with minimizing the role of the medical history, 1:1 patient interview, etc.

PEARL: Remember what has been repeated often in this book—RATING SCALES ARE SCREENING TOOLS. THEY ARE AIDS TO DIAGNOSIS BUT OF ARE NOT DIAGNOSTIC BY THEMSELVES.

3. Diagnosing and treating complex medical conditions, such as ADHD and autism, and developmental disabilities, along with chronic problems including asthma, diabetes, and epilepsy, can be very challenging and require the utmost in communication skills and TRUST among the patient, family, and physician.

PEARL: The more we delegate the information we receive for treatment recommendations to either online entrees or patient handouts, we sacrifice the patient-physician trust relationship that is necessary for optimal care.

ADDITIONAL HELPFUL LOCAL RESOURCES FOR THE PRIMARY CARE CLINICIAN SEEING MENTAL HEALTH

1. Organize a small group (5—8) of your fellow clinicians and meet once or twice monthly (1 h in the morning before starting to see patients).
   - "Pick each other's brains" regarding challenging cases.
   - It is true "two heads are better than one."
   - It will improve both your diagnostic and therapeutic acumen.
2. Once in a month consider a catered lunch for a similar purpose but include ancillary personnel from the local community, such as child psychiatry, school counseling and/or school psychology, ADHD coaching, and special education. Discuss anonymously one or two complex cases.

   There are several benefits to this approach:
   - It facilitates discussion of other diagnoses and treatments, perhaps not considered by you.
   - It is a great education exercise to hear a case discussed from a different specialty viewpoint.
   - It helps develop collegial relationships with other specialties in the school and community, which can be very helpful in managing complex issues. When referrals are needed, "it is always great to know and respect the person at the other end of the line."

   Note: Both the abovementioned recommendations could be done digitally, e.g., via Skype.
3. If possible develop a collegial relationship with a fellow child/adolescent psychiatrist in your community who could be available for urgent psychiatric consultations, or even urgent phone consult to you regarding a worrisome, perhaps suicidal patient, serious side effect to medications, etc. (Some communities have a resource phone line available to the community clinicians, e.g., the PAL system at the Seattle Children's Hospital, for emergency phone consultation regarding urgent psychiatric issues.)

HELPFUL OFFICE TECHNIQUES IN EVALUATION AND FOLLOW-UP OF ADHD IN CHILDREN AND ADOLESCENTS

1. Put a staff person (e.g., medical assistant) in charge of all the intake issues (e.g., receiving the referrals, making sure all the paperwork is organized, sending out and receiving the packets from families, teachers), obtaining other information (school or private evaluations, etc.), and then making the appropriate appointments.

This person would also make follow-up appointments, making sure that rating scales from parents and teachers are received prior to each appointment.

Give this person a responsible title, such as "ADHD coordinator," to enhance prestige and importance (it works!). This system also greatly improves consistency and efficiency of the whole appointment process.

2. **PEARL:** If possible make teacher rating scales, questionnaires, etc., able to be completed online and emailed to the clinic. This greatly enhances compliance, along with ensuring more informed clinical decision-making. However privacy needs to be ensured.
3. Always spend some one-to-one time with adolescents during follow-up appointments (may then see parents alone, if needed, or together with the adolescent). Also, never seeing parents in follow-up visits is not conducive sometimes of obtaining an accurate assessment as to how things are going. An occasional private visit with a high-school patient who is compliant with treatment, stable, and doing well as per school reports, etc., can be very appropriate on a case-by-case basis, particularly if the visit is supplemented by a brief phone call report from the parent. College-aged students are obviously often seen alone.
4. In middle school/high school, rating scales from teachers may not be as helpful as progress reports, as teacher ability is hampered by the large number of students taught and the lack of specific behavioral observation needed to complete the form. Progress reports should denote test results, homework completion, grades, etc.
5. Be very thorough about obtaining height, weight, and blood pressure at each follow-up appointment. Also plot these carefully on a growth chart. Losing weight is not unusual on stimulant medication, but weight gain is essential to ensure normal growth in height. Falling away from the normal height percentile is not acceptable and must be assessed and remedied. (Is it due to the current medicine or another factor?)
6. It is recommended to screen all adolescents at least yearly for anxiety and/or depression, using the SCARED and PHQ-9 questionnaires, respectively, or a proven proprietary rating scale. Also, whenever things deteriorate repeat screening would be appropriate, even when symptoms are not clearly evident or minimal. If coexisting conditions, such as anxiety or depression, are diagnosed and treated, serial rating scales can be very helpful in demonstrating the response to treatment.

7. The same approach is very helpful in monitoring for substance abuse, e.g., using the CRAFFT screening tool. USE THIS SCREENING TOOL OFTEN IN ADOLESCENTS.
8. Sudden or even more gradual deterioration of ADHD symptom control, falling grades, or school behavior/problems should suggest several possibilities, including the following:
    a. Is the current medicine dose inadequate because of a growth spurt, or has it just lost its effectiveness?
    b. Is the patient noncompliant, or forgetful in taking it, perhaps when parents put the adolescent "in charge of his medications?"
    c. Has the adolescent become resistant to taking medications, perhaps by peer pressure, or spitting it out when parents are not observing?
    d. Has the adolescent developed anxiety or depression as a coexisting problem that needs evaluation and treatment?
    e. Has the patient succumbed to substance abuse, e.g., smoking pot, which has caused the ADHD to deteriorate?

There are even other possibilities. It is urgent to get to the bottom of what is going on and to get appropriate responses in place.

PEARL: Adolescents often say, "My friends don't like me when I take my meds" (often because they no longer are as funny, such as blurting out inappropriate comments).

GUIDELINES FOR ADHD MEDICATION PRESCRIPTIONS AND REFILLS

1. Medication refills are a major opportunity to monitor the behavior and academic progress of children and adolescents with ADHD.
2. Refills should never be automatic without ascertaining the information in the following list. This basically means a phone interview of the parent/caretaker by the healthcare provider's office (presumably an RN) every month.

PEARL: As stimulant medications are controlled drugs and cannot be refilled without a new prescription, it encourages/forces the abovementioned scenario to occur, i.e., monthly phone calls to the clinician office.

This is time-consuming and might be considered a "hassle" by both the parent and the clinician. Nonetheless, our experience with literally thousands of patients has shown it is the best way to ensure optimal control of symptoms and medication response.

In the case of nonstimulant ADHD medications, such as α-agonists or atomoxetine, automatic monthly refills should be limited to three to four times to correspond to the check-back appointments every 3—4 months. Automatic refills for 6—12 months are an invitation for poor or uncontrolled management of ADHD symptoms and treatment.

This type of monitoring is crucial to provide optimal care. Deterioration in performance can occur fairly quickly (e.g., growth spurt, noncompliance in taking medications) and needs to be checked immediately or proactively rather than 3 months later.

PEARL: The Multimodal Treatment Study of Children with ADHD (MTA) showed that less frequent monitoring in the control group (community MD care) resulted in less optimal response to medications than the study group.

3. Important information to remember:
    • The average child with ADHD requires a dosage change once or twice yearly (due to growth, increasing stress of school, etc.).
    • Research (e.g., MTA) shows that to provide optimal care and response to medications, three to four check-back appointments to the clinician are required yearly.
    • Phone voicemail comments by the parent to the clinician office, such as "everything is fine," do not hold up under scrutiny. The use of rating scales (e.g., teacher and parent follow-up Vanderbilt questionnaires) is necessary for accurate assessment, particularly the teacher form.

PEARL: In middle school and high school where teachers have large numbers of students (e.g., math or English) and know the student less well than elementary teachers, the information on the monthly progress report might be more helpful. (If progress reports are not routinely done by the school or teachers use a 504 plan to make that mandatory.)

PEARL: Some clinician offices have set up a secure phone line through which information such as rating scales and progress reports can be safely sent to the clinician's office.

THIS REALLY enhances the accuracy and VALUE of the follow-up system.

4. Each monthly phone visit to the clinician office should inquire about the following:
    • Behavior: School and home
    • Academic performance: Grades, tests, homework
    • Sleep: Insomnia, etc.
    • Appetite: Weight gain/loss, etc.
    • Side effects: Headache, stomachache, tics, lethargy, irritability, etc.

Based on the information from the phone call a decision is made by the clinician/office as to whether the medication and dosage are appropriate, other treatments are indicated, there is need for an urgent follow-up appointment, etc.

5. If the child has not been seen by the clinician for 3–4 months the parent will be informed at the time of refill that no subsequent refills will be given until the child is seen. If possible make a return appointment for the child then. In some instances, it might be necessary to give only a limited number of pills, e.g., for 10–14 days, pending an urgent return appointment.

6. If a child's medication dosage is increased because of increased ADHD symptoms, or an abnormal Vanderbilt questionnaire, a follow-up rating scale or questionnaire should be obtained in 2–4 weeks to show improvement in symptoms and performance.

PEARL: Remember that medications improve core ADHD symptoms but do not necessarily improve executive function, so that completing homework may need other accommodations and/or training, e.g., study skills, tutoring, mentoring, homework club.

7. In general, medications should be given 365 days per year. The only really valid exception to not taking medications on weekends, holidays, and vacations is when the child really struggles to gain weight. In that situation, medication-free days may be a great help or even a necessity (some parents refuse to follow this rule, e.g., routinely discontinuing the medication for the summer). Being flexible about this and having an open discussion with the parents and child, leading hopefully to a joint decision, works the best (sometimes a smaller dose works well, given the less demand on the child's attentional needs, or medication can be given only when the child goes to camp or attends summer school).

8. In adolescents exposed to risk behavior or who are driving, taking medication 365 days per year is overwhelmingly supported by research (e.g., unmedicated drivers with ADHD are three to four times more likely to have an accident than their peers without ADHD).

PEARL: Parents should have a "tough-love" approach. "IF YOU WANT TO DRIVE, YOU TAKE YOUR MEDICATIONS. NO EXCEPTIONS!"

9. In the first 2–4 weeks of starting a new medication, transient symptoms such as headache, stomach ache, decreased appetite, or mild weight loss are common. Parents and children/adolescents should be encouraged to minimize the symptoms that are usually transient.

PEARL: It is very important for the clinician to proactively discuss with the parent and child/adolescent about these potential side effects and also to promptly deal with symptoms to lessen the possibility of noncompliance or cessation of medication.

10. Appetite loss for lunch is common and expected (medicine peak effect). Parents are encouraged to push healthy snacks after school and at bedtime, e.g., breakfast drinks, milk shakes.

PEARL: Consultation with a nutritionist is often very helpful to increase calorie intake.

11. Sleep issues (insomnia) should first be treated with good sleep habits such as
    • bedtime routine,
    • turning off all electronics (especially cell phones, computers, etc.) 30 min prior to bedtime,
    • light music OK if helpful,
    • snacking,
    • light reading.

12. If these are not successful then consider
    • melatonin, 5–6 mg, 30 min prior to bedtime (or Benadryl, 25 mg);
    • change to an 8-h medication;
    • trial of clonidine, 0.1–0.2 mg, 30 min before bedtime (or long-acting α-agonist);
    • try a nonstimulant, such as atomoxetine at bedtime.

13. Persistent sleep issues, particularly when symptoms of sleep deprivation are noted (e.g., falling asleep in class), then consider other interventions:
    • Rule out excessive caffeine intake, coffee, energy drinks
    • Sleep study/consult sleep disorder specialist
    • Assess for coexistent disorders, e.g., anxiety or depression
    • Trial of trazodone
    • Consult psychiatry

14. Stimulant medication might make a patient without ADHD jittery or agitated, whereas a patient with ADHD often has a paradoxically opposite reaction: too large a dose may cause the child/adolescent to feel "flat," "sluggish," or "like a zombie."

PEARL: This is a particularly intolerant side effect of adolescent patients with ADHD, and if not recognized and treated by lowering the dosage, the result will be refusal to take the medication or noncompliance.

ORGANIZING AN ADHD PARENT TRAINING COURSE

Purpose: To equip parents of children and adolescents with ADHD to provide the best environment for the child to progress through childhood and adolescence and become a functional adult. (This model was developed at The Center for ADHD, Seattle, in 1989, and was used to train hundreds of parent couples. It became a national model.)

Format

- Six to ten parent couples
- Topic presentation and discussion
- When: Evenings, 2 h one evening/week, for 8 weeks
- Cost: Flexible, e.g., $10 per couple per session, liberal use of scholarships (e.g., for single parents)
- Where: Usually clinic waiting room, or classroom in school, church, local agency, etc.
- Staff: Mostly educational or healthcare professionals knowledgeable in child development, education, ADHD, e.g., nurse practitioners, family therapists, school counselors (usually MD or pediatric nurse practitioner to present discussion about medications).

Agenda

Class 1, overview of ADHD: History, symptoms, diagnosis, multimodal treatments, outcomes, coexistent problems, etc. Resources include books, websites, etc. (see subsequent chapter 18 on parent resources.).
Classes 2–4, behavior therapy for ADHD
- Examples:
  Behavior modification techniques
  Reward/consequence systems
  Time out
  Token economies
  Daily report card
- 1-2-3 Magic (workbook and video), a technique developed by Tom Phelan, PhD, which is quite effective for preadolescent children with ADHD.
- Contracts for adolescents
- Homework regarding the abovementioned techniques for parents to try, report back to class, etc.
Class 5, educational rights and supports available and necessary for kids with ADHD
- Individuals with Disabilities Education Act: Special education if delays in achievement, need for tutoring, other interventions (occupational therapy, physical therapy, etc.)
- 504 Plans: Other accommodations, e.g., extra time for tests, preferential seating, to lessen discrimination and ensure academic success

- Choosing a teacher, how to monitor school progress, homework completion, etc.
- Outside agencies to help, e.g., tutoring
- College preparation and selection
Class 6, medications: Uses, success rate, side effects, risks, etc. (taught by MD, e.g., pediatrician or nurse practitioner). Also abuse, diversion of medications.
Class 7, coexistent problems (e.g., anxiety, depression, substance abuse)
- How to monitor emotional health (screening tools)
- How to diagnose and treat (anxiety, depression)
- Issues regarding alcohol, pot, etc.
Class 8, summary items
- Advocacy for your child (school, sports, social/peer groups, etc.)
- Vocational goals, expectations
- Adult ADHD: Discussion regarding any parents in group who realize they had or have ADHD, where/how they could receive help
An optional opportunity is to attend an online course, such as the one mentioned earlier, is through the CHADD organization ("Parent to Parent Program"). See www.chadd.org.

SETTING UP A QUALITY IMPROVEMENT PROJECT IN YOUR PRACTICE FOR ADHD CARE (OR OTHER MENTAL HEALTH DIAGNOSIS)

Read July 2016 *Pediatrics* (Jeff Epstein, et al.).

Using a technology-assisted intervention (ADHD Care Quality software) improved the ADHD care quality and resulted in additional reductions in parent-rated ADHD symptoms among patients prescribed with ADHD medications.

Many clinics and practice settings are beginning to set up Quality Improvement (QI) projects around some aspect of patient care. This can be very rewarding for at least two reasons. First, it will show that in doing so you are really demonstrating that you are improving care to your patients. Even if it is not monumental or earth-shattering, it will enhance your satisfaction with what you are doing. Second, many of these types of QI projects will be accepted by the American Board of Pediatrics (ABP) as evidence of fulfilling certain recertification requirements. (ABP has their own program you can join.)

Suppose you set up a simple goal like this. "At least 90% of my adolescents diagnosed with ADHD will be screened at least once yearly for depression." This could be entered into the clinic procedures where the receptionist could have the chart flagged as to the need for the adolescent to complete the PHQ-9 when they come in for the next appointment. Sounds simple, and it can be, but it fulfills one of the major goals this book has talked about, namely, to screen high-risk adolescents at least yearly for depression, even if they do not have symptoms anyone has observed. How satisfying it is as a clinician to identify such an unmet need in an adolescent and arrange treatment accommodations rather than seeing the adolescent down the road when things in his or her life have spiraled downward!

Motivational Interviewing

What is motivational interviewing (MI)?

The AAP defines it as (paraphrased) an interview technique designed to motivate the patient to change health behavior. The goal of MI is to involve the patient in the problem-solving process. It is basically a "conversation about change," rather than the clinician just giving advice as we so often do.

Current scenario: Doctor says, "John you need to lose 35#. You might have a heart attack." John says, "Yeah I know. I've tried before but nothing helps."

MI scenario: Doctor says, "John, I notice your weight has been creeping up the last few years. Would you be willing to talk about that?" John says, "Sure."

The following mnemonic is helpful in guiding the interview: "LEAP"

L—Listen (active listening), open-ended questions

E—Empathize, educate, encourage

A—Agree. Find areas you and patient agree on to start the process of change

P—Partner, plan, proceed

The following is a collaborative discussion with John about possibilities, and hopes, for change. MI can be used to empower the patient to assume desire and responsibility for making change.

The following techniques, among others, are often utilized:

1. Using open-ended questions
2. Being empathetic and supportive
3. Being nonjudgmental
4. Being nondictatorial
5. Discussing pros and cons of making changes
6. Discussing the importance of making changes
7. Summarizing

Does it work? Current evidence suggests it can be very helpful in counseling on substance abuse, smoking, diet/weight loss, exercise, and possibly anxiety and depression. AAP feels MI has been found to be more effective than no treatment, and in many cases more effective than other treatments. Furthermore, MI is also believed to be more cost-effective than other treatments.

Myth: "Takes a lot of time." In fact, it can be utilized in very brief encounters with patients, once the technique is learned.

Reference: Google for AAP/MI. Many links are provided to simulated interviews, on how to learn the technique, etc.

Another helpful website is http.www.motivationalinterviewing.org.

This website is for the Motivational Interviewing Network of Trainers, which provides 1-day training sessions at locations throughout the United States.

Understanding Cultural Diversity in Mental Health Issues

In the recent years, particularly with the influx of many new ethnic groups into the United States, we have become increasingly aware of cultural differences in customs, clothing, religion, mores, vocational aspirations and dreams, etc. Along with these cultural differences, disparities in healthcare, particularly mental healthcare, have appeared. As clinicians who deliver mental healthcare, it is important that we become thoroughly acquainted with these disparities so that our caregiving will not only be evidence-based but also be made acceptable to the patients of various ethnicities for whom we care.

There are two publications that will give us an understanding of these disparities and provide some guidance to us as we interact with our patients of varying cultures.

1. Margarita Alegria, et al. *Child and Adolescent Psychiatric Clinics of North America* 19(4):759–774, October 2010.

This is an excellent and very comprehensive review article that describes the current status of mental healthcare in the United States and the racial and ethnic disparities in both diagnosis and provision of treatment.

2. Practice parameter for cultural competence in child and adolescent psychiatric practice. It was published by the *Journal of the American Academy of Child and Adolescent Psychiatry* in December 2013 and lists 13 helpful principles for clinicians providing mental health treatment to ethnic and racial minority groups (direct quotations are in quotes and my comments are in parentheses).

Principle 1. "Clinicians should identify and address barriers (economic, geographic, insurance, cultural beliefs, stigma, etc.) that may prevent culturally diverse children and their families from obtaining mental health services." (e.g., Non-Hispanic Whites are much more accepting of mental health services than some minority groups because of such things as stigma, cost, transportation, language.)

Principle 2. "Clinicians should conduct the evaluation in the language in which the child and family are proficient." (by using interpreters who are skilled and trained and, e.g., questionnaires in the language of the patient/family)

Principle 3. "Clinicians should understand the impact of dual-language competence on the child's adaptation and functioning." (Do not readily recommend the discontinuation of the home language, which may result in negative consequences.)

Principle 4. "Clinicians should be cognizant that cultural biases might interfere with their clinical judgement, and work toward addressing these biases." (to assure equality)

Principle 5. "Clinicians should apply knowledge of cultural differences in developmental progression, idiomatic expressions of distress, and symptomatic presentation for different disorders, to the clinical formulation and diagnosis." (Sometimes, these different symptomatic presentations may be wrongly misinterpreted as a psychopathologic condition.)

Resource: The Cultural Formulation Interview. A 16-item semistructured interview to obtain information about the impact of culture on clinical presentation and care, with suggested questions to inquire about different domains.

Principle 6. "Clinicians should assess for an immigration-related loss or trauma and community trauma (violence, abuse) in the child and family and address these concerns in the treatment." (e.g., separation, torture, detention)

Principle 7. "Clinicians should evaluate and address in treatment the acculturation level, and presence of acculturation stress, and intergenerational acculturation on family conflict in diverse children and families." (The conflict between how one sees oneself within the family vs. how one sees oneself in the new culture.)

Principle 8. "Clinicians should make special efforts to include family members, and key members of traditional extended families, such as grandparents or other elders, in the assessment, treatment planning, and treatment."

Principle 9. "Clinicians should evaluate and incorporate cultural strengths (including values, beliefs, and attitudes) in their treatment interventions, to enhance the child's and family's participation in treatment and its effectiveness."

Principle 10. "Clinicians should treat culturally diverse children and their families in familiar settings within their communities whenever possible." (e.g., school or neighborhood)

Principle 11. "Clinicians should support parents to develop appropriate behavioral management skills consonant with their cultural values and beliefs." (presuming none of these are illegal or incongruent with the new culture)

Principle 12. "Clinicians should preferentially use evidence-based psychological and pharmacologic interventions specific for the ethnic/racial population of the child and family they are serving." (e.g., using cognitive behavior therapy for the treatment of depression in the Hispanic patient, which has evidence base for this ethnic group.)

Principle 13 "Clinicians should identify ethnopharmacologic factors (pharmacogenomics, dietary, use of herbal cures) that may influence the child's response to medications, or experience of side-effects." (e.g., African Americans do not respond as well to selective serotonin reuptake inhibitors, or may have more side effects, such as extrapyramidal symptoms, to the atypical antipsychotics or Asians may metabolize Western medicines more slowly and have increased side effects.)

PEARL: Often, neither these patients nor their American counterparts volunteer the information on the use of herbal or traditional medicines, which may either counteract Western medications or increase toxicity. It is imperative to ask for this information.

Mental Health Diagnoses Commonly Associated With Other Specific Medical/ Mental Health Conditions (Comorbidities)

1. **ADHD**: Oppositional defiant disorder, conduct disorder, anxiety, depression, aggression, obsessive-compulsive disorder, bipolar disorder, substance abuse disorder, learning disabilities
2. **Autistic spectrum**: ADHD symptoms, anxiety, obsessive-compulsive disorder, ritualism, aggression
3. **Bipolar disorder**: ADHD, anxiety, oppositional defiant disorder, conduct disorder, substance abuse disorder, migraine, intermittent explosive disorder, suicidal ideation/attempt

4. **Depression**: Anxiety, substance abuse disorder, obsessive-compulsive disorder, anorexia nervosa, bulimia, borderline personality disorder
5. **Disruptive mood dysregulation disorder:** Oppositional defiant disorder, mood/anxiety disorders
6. **Anxiety disorder**: Specific phobia, panic disorder, generalized anxiety disorder, substance abuse disorder, obsessive-compulsive disorder, bipolar disorder, depression
7. **Obsessive-compulsive disorder:** Anxiety disorder (panic, phobias), depression, bipolar disorder, posttraumatic stress disorder, trichotillomania, excoriation (skin), oppositional defiant disorder, eating disorders, Tourette syndrome
8. **Gender dysphoria (Lesbian/Bisexual/Transgender/ Queer [LBTJQ]):** Anxiety, depression, suicidal ideation/intent, disruptive and impulse control disorders, obesity, high-risk behavior
9. **Fragile X:** ADHD symptoms, aggression, learning disabilities
10. **Traumatic brain injury**: (e.g., near drowning), ADHD symptoms, aggression, learning disabilities
11. **Reactive attachment disorder:** ADHD symptoms, obsessive-compulsive disorder (hoarding)

PEARL: Remember, when assessing any of these mental health issues, the potential comorbidities must always be considered because they might be of more significance than the diagnosis itself, e.g., substance abuse, suicidality.

Implementing Mental Health Priorities in Practice—Strategies to Engage Patients and Families

PEARL: These are great videos produced by the AAP (in 2016) to engage patients and families and start discussion between caregivers and families about mental health concerns. Make use of them! The videos are available for purchase from the AAP, for viewing by patients and families, with the intent of focusing further discussions of subjects discussed on the videos.

1. Introduction
2. Motivational Interviewing
3. Social and emotional problems
4. Depression
5. Inattention and impulsivity
6. Disruptive behavior and aggression
7. Substance abuse
8. Self-harm and suicide

CHAPTER 18

ADHD Resources for Clinicians, Parents, and Patients

BOOKS (FOR PARENTS, CLINICIANS, AND EDUCATORS)

Russell Barkley. Taking charge of ADHD, 3rd Ed., 2013.

Joyce Cooper-Kahn. Late, lost, and unprepared. (Executive function skills).

Chris Dendy. Teenagers with ADD and ADHD, 2nd Ed.

Sandra Rief. The ADHD book of lists, 2nd Ed. (Educational Helps).

Kathleen Nadeau, Ellen Littman, and Patricia Quinn. Understanding girls with ADHD, 2nd Ed., 2015.

Kathleen Nadeau. Survival guide for college students with ADHD or LD, 2nd Ed.

AAP. ADHD: a complete and authoritative guide, 2nd Ed.

Mark Wolraich and George DuPaul. ADHD diagnosis and management: a practical guide for the clinic and classroom, 2010.

Russell Barkley. Your defiant child, 2nd Ed., 2013.

Ross W. Green. The explosive child, 2009.

Lynn Clark: SOS: Help for parents. (Ages 2—12.) Improving behavior and emotional adjustment of children.

Matthew Cohen. A guide to special education advocacy, 2009 (Legal Rights).

Chris Zeigler Dendy and Mary Durheim. CHADD educators manual, www.chadd.org.

CHADD information and resource guide, 2nd Ed., www.chadd.org (for parents of children with ADHD).

Peter Jensen. Making the system work for your child with ADHD, 2004, The Guilford Press.

Ari Tuckman. More attention, less deficit. Success strategies for adults with ADHD.

Robert Brooks and Sam Goldstein. Raising resilient children, McGraw Hill.

Tamar E. Chansky. Freeing your child from anxiety, Three Rivers Press.

WEBSITES: ADHD/LEARNING DISABILITY, MENTAL HEALTH, PARENTING, BEHAVIORAL ISSUES IN CHILDREN

The Incredible Years, http://incredibleyears.com/.

Triple P, www.triplep.net.

Parent-Child Interaction Therapy, www.pcit.org.

Google: The Coping Cat Program. A CBT workbook program for children with Anxiety.

Google: International OCD Foundation. Parent resource for children with OCD.

Google: The National Sleep Foundation and Sleep Diary. Websites regarding sleep issues.

www.AnxietyBC.com. Resources for parents and caregivers regarding anxiety.

Google: Trans Youth Family Allies. Information on transgender youth.

Google: World Professional Association for Transgender Health (WPATH). Educational organization on transgender health.

www.drugs@fda.org. Search for medications by name and read about side effects, etc.

www.thereachinstitute.org. Read the REACH Newsletter article entitled "Is my child getting CBT?"

Google: "Find A CBT Therapist" (by zip code).

www.add.org, ADDA (Attention Deficit Disorder Association).

www.chadd.org, CHADD organization.

www.help4adhd.org, National Resource Center for ADHD.

www.adhd.com, ADHD Family Support Center.

www.addwarehouse.com, ADD Warehouse— available written resources for ADHD.

www.aap.org, American Academy of Pediatrics (search ADHD).

www.aacap.org, American Academy of Child and Adolescent Psychiatry (search Family Resources).

www.mayoclinic.org (search ADHD).

http://www.sandrarief.com, Sandra Rief is a nationally recognized educator for ADHD/learning disability.

www.ncld.org, National Center for Learning Disabilities.

www.nichd.nih.gov, National Institute of Child Health and Child Development (search ADHD).

www.nimh.nih.gov, National Institute of Mental Health (search ADHD).

www.ldanatl.org, Learning Disabilities Association of America (LDA).

www.parentsmedguide.org, (AACAP) Practical information on ADHD, pediatric depression, and bipolar disorder.

www.bpkids.org, Child and Adolescent Bipolar Foundation.

www.dbsalliance.org, Depression and Bipolar Support Alliance.

www.ffcmh.org, Federation of Families for Children's Mental Health.

www.nami.org, National Alliance on Mental Illness.

www.nmha.org, National Mental Health Association.

www.dbpeds.org, Section on Developmental/Behavioral Pediatrics (AAP). It contains material on child development, behavior and emotional screening, parent handouts, and information on other mental health websites.

EVIDENCE-BASED PARENT BEHAVIOR PROGRAMS FOR CHILDREN/ ADOLESCENTS WITH ADHD

1. Triple P (Positive Parenting Program), www.triplep.net.[a]
2. The Incredible Years Parenting Program, www.incredibleyears.com.[a]
3. Parent-Child Interaction Therapy, www.pcit.org.[a]
4. New Forest Parenting Program (Google name).[a]
5. STAR Parenting Program (Google name).
6. Strengthening Families Program (Google name).
7. Community Parent Education Program (COPE) (Google name).
8. Parent Management Training Institute (Google name).
9. Training Parents as Friendship Coaches (Google University of British Columbia's Peer Relationships in Childhood Lab).
10. Systematic Training for Effective Parenting (STEP), www.steppublishers.com.
11. Helping the Noncompliant Child, www.cebc4cw.org.[a]
12. CHADD: Parent to Parent Family Training on ADHD, www.chadd.org.

[a] Applicable to preschool children.

BOOKS FOR CHILDREN AND ADOLESCENTS (EXAMPLES), AVAILABLE AT ADD WAREHOUSE (WWW.ADDWAREHOUSE.COM)

ADHD in the young child (ages 3–6 years).

Eukee the jumpy, jumpy elephant (ages 5–7 years).

Slam dunk: a young boy's struggle with ADD (ages 8–12 years).

Some kids just can't sit still! (ages 4–9 years).

Making the grade (ages 9–14 years).

Problem solver guide for students with ADHD (adolescents).

Behavior training (manual and video, preadolescent), Tom Phelan, PhD (1-2-3 magic program).

ADDITIONAL BIBLIOGRAPHY FOR CLINICIANS

A. ADHD

1. Schoenfelder E, Kollins S. ADHD and health-risk behaviors: toward prevention and health promotion. *J Pediatr Psychol.* 2016;41(7):735–740. This is a good review article of risk behaviors (such as substance abuse, smoking, obesity/binge eating, unsafe sexual activity, violence, accidents, reduced socioeconomic attainment, and quality of life). It discusses multimodality care in prevention, screening, and treatment.
2. Pliszka SR, Crismon ML, et al. CMAP algorithms for the pharmacological treatment of ADHD, with a) comorbid anxiety disorder, b) comorbid aggression, and c) comorbid tic disorder. *J Am Acad Child Adolesc Psychiatry.* 2006;45:642–657. **PEARL:** It provides excellent algorithms for medication treatment of complex ADHD, e.g., when coexistent confounding conditions are present, including anxiety, aggression, tics, etc. (These algorithms have become the STANDARD OF CARE.) See examples of how they should work in the Scenario section of ADHD Treatment (chapter 4).
3. McCabe SE, et al. Age of onset, duration, and type of medication therapy for ADHD, and substance abuse during adolescence: a multi-cohort national study. *J Am Acad Child Adolesc Psychiatry.* 2016;55(6):479–486. A total of 40,358 individuals from 10 cohorts (2005–14), including 52% women, 62% white, 10% African Americans, 14% Hispanic, and 14% others. Individuals who initiated stimulant therapy later (age 10–14 years, and 15 years and older)

and for shorter duration (2 years or less, and 3—5 years) as well as those who reported only nonstimulant medication therapy for ADHD had significantly greater odds of substance abuse in adolescence relative to individuals who initiated stimulant medication therapy earlier (age 9 years or less) and for longer duration. **PEARL:** We have long known that untreated adolescents with ADHD have three to four times greater incidence of substance abuse than those without ADHD, and it can be quite devastating. HOW TO POSSIBLY PREVENT ADOLESCENT SUBSTANCE ABUSE? DIAGNOSE ADHD EARLY, BEFORE AGE 9 YEARS, AND TREAT WITH STIMULANTS IF POSSIBLE (NOT NON-STIMULANTS) THROUGH ADOLESCENCE!

4. J. Swanson, et al. Young adult outcomes in the follow-up of the multimodal treatment study of attention-deficit/hyperactivity disorder: symptom persistence, source discrepancy, and height suppression. *J Child Psychol Psychiatry*, 10 March 2017.

This a follow-up study of the original MTA study published in 1999 of a 14-month randomized control study of 579 children with ADHD, aged 7—10 years, who were subjected to medication treatment, behavior therapy, and combined therapy, and it included a control group as well (see the section Hallmark Research Studies Every Clinician Should Review). Of the original 579 cases, 515 were consented for continuation and were compared in this current study to 289 classmates as controls (258 without ADHD). Results: (1) Those patients (somewhat less in number) who continued medicine treatment into adulthood showed no difference in severity of symptoms compared with those who had intermittent breaks in treatment (e.g., drug holidays), or who discontinued taking medications altogether. (2) The average height of those who continued treatment into adulthood was about 2 cm shorter than those who did not continue treatment.

Authors of the study concluded "Childhood-onset ADHD is a chronic disorder with persistence of symptoms into adulthood, ... and extended use of stimulant medications from childhood through adolescence is associated with a mild suppression (1") of adult height but is not associated with reduced symptom severity."

This provocative report, admittedly based on a relatively small sample, raises many unanswered questions regarding the nature of ADHD, its chronicity, and what, as of now, unknown factors contribute to successful or unsuccessful outcomes.

5. Divorsky M. and Langberg J. A review of factors that promote resilience in youth with ADHD and ADHD symptoms. *Clin Child Fam Psychol Rev.* 2016;19:368—391. doi:10.1007/s10567-016-0216-z.

This is a review of the studies in the medical literature regarding resilience in youth with ADHD or ADHD symptoms ($n = 21$ studies). Conclusion: Resilience is defined as "positive patterns of adaptation in the context of adversity." "Overall there was solid evidence for social acceptance as protective in youth with ADHD. There was also compelling evidence supporting positive parenting as a promoting factor...the study of other individual, family, and social mechanisms remains in its infancy." (needs more research).

B. Antipsychotic medications
   1. Correll CU, Carlson HE. Endocrine and metabolic adverse effects of psychotropic medications in children and adolescents. *J Am Acad Child Adolesc Psychiatry*. 2006;45:771—791.
   2. Liv HY, Potter MP, Woodward Y, et al. Pharmacologic treatments for pediatric bipolar disorder: a review and meta-analysis. *J Am Acad Child Adolesc Psychiatry*. 2011;50(8).
C. Suicide
   1. Sheftall A, et al. Suicide in elementary school-aged children and early adolescents. *Pediatrics*. 2016:138(4):e20160436. (A review of national data 2003—2012 for 17 US states, including 693 patients aged 5—14 years.)
   2. Nock M, et al. Prevalence, correlates, and treatment of lifetime suicidal behavior among adolescents: results from the National Comorbidity Survey Replication Adolescent Supplement. *JAMA Psychiatry*. Published Online January 9, 2013. www.JAMAPSYCH.com.
D. Aggression
   1. Treatment of maladaptive aggression in youth (T-MAY). Results from a consensus survey of experts—recommended best practices. See also chapter 14, re: Aggressive Child.
   2. Pappadopulos E, et al. *J Child Adolesc Psychopharmacol*. 2011;21:505—515.

E. Mental health in children

AAP Technical Report. Gleason M, et al. Addressing early childhood emotional and behavioral problems. *Pediatrics*. 2016;138(6):e20163025.

This is an excellent thorough report of a task force summarizing the status in the United States regarding mental health of children and adolescents and the need for not only more community resources but also more involvement by primary care clinicians (pediatricians) in early interventional diagnosis and treatment.

Resources for parents include the following:

The Incredible Years, http://incredibleyears.com.

Triple P, www.triplep.net.

Parent-Child Interaction Therapy, www.pcit.org.

F. Listing of practice parameters of the American Academy of Child and Adolescent Psychiatry (posttraumatic stress disorder, autism, atypical antipsychotic medication, cultural competency, eating disorders, reactive attachment disorder, etc.).

https://www.aacap.org/AACAP/Resources_for_ Primary_Care/Practice_Parameters_and_Resource_ Centers/Practice_Parameters.aspx.

G. Mental health emergencies

Chun TH, et al. AAP Committee on Emergency Medicine. Executive summary: evaluation and management of children with acute mental health or behavioral problems. Part I: common clinical challenges of patients with mental health and/or behavioral emergencies. *Pediatrics*. 2016; 138(3).

Chun TH, et al. AAP Committee on Emergency Medicine. Executive summary: Part II: recognition of clinically challenging mental health related conditions presenting with medical or uncertain symptoms. *Pediatrics*. 2016;138(3): e20161574.

H. Depression in adolescents (http://www.reachout 4teens.org)

"Reaching Out to Adolescents in Distress" (ROAD) is a joint study by the Seattle Children's Hospital, Group Health Cooperative, and University of Washington.

This is an interesting and provocative study of a collaborative care intervention, involving a case manager based in a primary care setting, who provided education to depressed adolescents and their parents, arranged CBT therapy, and worked with the MD to initiate antidepressant medication. The case manager met weekly with the patient and observed response to therapy, and if there was a lack of response, the case manager provided more

intensive therapy per a protocol. After a year, teens receiving collaborative care were three times more likely to have received evidence-based therapy, had greater decrease in depression symptoms, and had more than twice as much remission of depression compared with "routine care."

Richardson LP, et al. Collaborative care for adolescents with depression in primary care: a randomized clinical trial. *JAMA*, August 2014.

Question: Integrating mental health into practices. Is this the future of primary care?

I. Sege RD. AAP Committee on Child Abuse and Neglect, Council on Foster Care, Adoption, and Kinship Care, American Academy of Child and Adolescent Psychiatry Committee on Child Maltreatment and Violence, National Center for Child Traumatic Stress. Clinical considerations related to the behavioral manifestations of child maltreatment. *Pediatrics*. 2017;139(4).

It is a follow-up extensive report, from an original report in 2008, of children who have experienced traumatic events, including abuse and neglect.

This report further guides the pediatrician in recognizing and managing the behavioral and mental health symptoms exhibited by maltreated children and in seeking appropriate therapy to help affected children in ways that may mitigate the consequences of child maltreatment.

The most trauma-specific psychiatric diagnosis associated with child maltreatment is posttraumatic stress disorder. Other issues commonly associated are internalizing problems (anxiety, depression) and externalizing problems (oppositional defiant disorder, conduct disorder, substance abuse, suicidal behavior, and ADHD signs and symptoms).

This is a summary of all the issues comprising diagnosis and treatment of children who have experienced child maltreatment and should be read by all primary care clinicians who treat children.

J. Tom Boat, Marshal Land, and Laurel Leslie. Healthcare workforce development to enhance mental and behavioral health of children and youth. *JAMA Pediatr*. 2017:171(11):1031–1032.

Recent report from a joint AAP/ABP task force.

K. Kotte A, et al. Autistic traits in children with and without ADHD. *Pediatrics*. 2013;132:e612–e622.

"Conclusion: A substantial minority of ADHD children manifest Autistic Traits (ATs), and those exhibiting ATs have greater severity of illness and dysfunction."

Recent article on this topic: Gordon-Lipkin E, et al. *Pediatrics*, March 30, 2018. It is a follow-up of the topic of autistic traits in children with ADHD and describes the increased problem of anxiety and depression as comorbid conditions in these children with dual diagnoses.

L. Screening children and adolescents for trauma (physical, mental, sexual, accidental, environmental, etc.)

Helpful screening tools: Child and Adolescent Trauma Screen (CATS), caregiver questionnaire for children aged 3–17 years and adolescent self-report. Available for free online. Google Child and Adolescent Trauma Screen (CATS), then check Assessment-University of Washington.

Good resource: The National Child Traumatic Stress Network (NCTSN).

HALLMARK RESEARCH STUDIES EVERY CLINICIAN SHOULD REVIEW

1. A 14-month randomized clinical trial of treatment strategies for attention-deficit/hyperactivity disorder. The MTA Cooperative Group. Multimodal Treatment Study of Children with ADHD. *Arch Gen Psychiatry*. 1999;56:1073–1086.
2. March J, et al. Treatment of Adolescent Depression Study (TADS) Team. *JAMA*, August 2004.
3. Walkup J, et al. CAMS: (Childhood Anxiety Multimodal Study). *N Engl J Med*, October 2008.
4. Greenhill L, et al. PATS: (Preschool ADHD Treatment Study). *J Am Acad Child Adolesc Psychiatry*, November 2006.

THE ABOVE MENTIONED SHOULD BE REQUIRED READING FOR ALL CLINICIANS.

PARENT HANDOUTS
Enhancing Self-Esteem

There are many published articles and books on enhancing self-esteem, which will not be duplicated here.

Rather than that, it would be more appropriate to share some simple principles learned over many years working with children and adolescents with ADHD, who often suffer a great deal with poor self-esteem.

It is always, without apology, necessary and important to shower your child or adolescent with love, praise, and commendation, at least 10 times more often than criticism. But there is also something equally or more important.

PEARL: Children's and adolescents' self-esteem is markedly enhanced when they learn, through positive accomplishments in daily life, that they really can

accomplish their goals and desires. Then the rise in self-esteem follows naturally. So our real job as parents and caregivers is to not only praise and assure them of their inherent worth but also MAKE SURE THEY ACHIEVE SUCCESSES.

There are three major areas in an adolescent's life with special needs where failure and loss of self-esteem occur.

So these are the areas where we need to focus.

PEARLS: Academic achievement:
1. Make sure they have been tested and their weaknesses are thoroughly understood.
2. Advocate, e.g., with the school. Shorter assignments, all the homework helps mentioned in earlier chapters, tutoring, etc.
3. Liberal use of 504 accommodations (or Individuals with Disabilities Education Act [IDEA]) if appropriate.
4. Realistic goals, particularly educational and vocational (they may be smart enough for college, but want to be a wood worker; encourage the latter).

Social skills:
1. Set realistic goals. Maybe one or two friends are adequate and appropriate for your child (research says it can be). Your child maybe does not need a big group of friends.
2. Foster social development. Encourage him/her to bring a friend to your family outings, hikes, visits to museums, even dinners. Then reciprocate.
3. Encourage involvement in some of your child's narrow-minded activities, e.g., chess club, robot or science club. If that is his or her interest then that is probably where he or she will make a close friend.

Athletics: Many or most adolescents with special needs have coordination issues (exception, Michael Phelps).
1. Don't force them into organized sports. Choose nonteam activities, such as hiking, bike riding, martial arts, swimming, where they can be successful at their own pace (also, these activities could involve a friend).

All of these areas take effort in forethought, planning, and execution. But the reward in enhancing your child's self-esteem can be not only rewarding but also life-changing. Remember, you the parent are the best advocate for your child.

TIPS FOR PARENTING A CHILD OR AN ADOLESCENT WITH ADHD

Use as a parent handout.
1. Choose a physician for your child who is interested in, or knowledgeable about, ADHD. May need

some help from neighbors, friends, local organizations, such as CHADD, Learning Disabilities Association (see resource list), PTA.

2. Make sure your child has been thoroughly assessed and correctly diagnosed (discuss with your child's personal physician).

3. Make sure your child's assessment included ruling out possible coexisting problems, including learning disorders, anxiety, depression, oppositional defiant disorder, and conduct disorder.

4. Educate yourself thoroughly about ADHD.
   - Recommended books:
     Russell Barkley. Taking charge of ADHD.
     Chris Dendy. Teenagers with ADD/ADHD.
     American Academy of Pediatrics. ADHD: a complete and authoritative guide.
     Sandra Rief. ADHD book of lists.
   - Website: www.chadd.org (Children with ADHD).
   - Groups: Attend local CHADD group if available in your community.

5. Know and understand the two scientifically proven treatments for ADHD:
   - Behavior therapy, e.g., rewards and consequences, token economies, time-out.
   - FDA-approved specific medications (stimulants and nonstimulants).

6. Avoid unproven/disproven treatments, particularly those that are potentially unsafe:
   - chiropractic,
   - herbal/nutritional supplements,
   - non−FDA-approved medications,
   - energy or "focus"-type drinks,
   - restrictive diets,
   - megavitamins.

7. Make sure your child is monitored regularly (research shows a visit at least every 3−4 months to the clinician is needed for optimal care).

8. Monitoring should include checking growth (height and weight), blood pressure, pulse, school progress (academics and behavior), side effects to medication (appetite, sleep, etc.), and peer and family relationships.

9. Monitoring should include rating scales completed by parent(s) and teacher(s) to assure that the ADHD treatment is optimal.

10. For most children, medication works best if given 365 days per year. Occasional exceptions apply, particularly if weight gain or linear growth on medication is impacted.

11. Understand fully the educational laws that provide learning assistance for your child with ADHD, including IDEA and Section 504 (see Chapter 3).

12. Develop a relationship with your child's teacher and arrange weekly communication (email, voicemail, progress note, etc.) regarding how the week went.
    This is more difficult at the middle-school and high-school level. Sometimes there is a "homework hotline" to call in. What you need to know as a parent is whether all the assignments for the week were turned in. Perhaps simple progress notes can be sent home (sometimes homework was done but not turned in).

13. Learn how to advocate for your child, for example, teacher selection or class schedule (if possible), preferential seating, extra time for tests, projects. THIS IS WHY HAVING A 504 PLAN IS HELPFUL!
    - Remember, no one knows your child as well as you!
    - Some parents hire an advocate or coach to help provide this mediation service, especially if they are "burned out."

14. Consider forming a team of consultants available to you, either singly or as a group, to assess, monitor, and make recommendations as problems develop. Such a team might include the following:
    - Child's physician
    - School personnel (contact), for example, counselor, psychologist, teacher, nurse
    - Advocate
    - Coach (such as tutor, homework monitor)
    - Family counselor

15. Remember children/adolescents with ADHD mature more slowly, for example, 2−3 years or so behind their peers, so your 13-year-old child might really be functioning at a 10-year-old level. "That explains a lot," you'll say.

16. Have realistic expectations for your child. Although really smart, he/she might desire vocational training rather than college.

17. Be realistic about sports. Kids with ADHD, even the good athletes, often struggle with team sports. They might do better with martial arts, bike riding, or swimming.

18. Do not expect your child with ADHD to be something he or she is not. For example, two or three friends might be plenty for your child, rather than a large group.

19. Know that a deterioration in your child's ADHD control needs immediate assessment to rule out problems such as
    - the medication dose is outgrown,
    - noncompliance with taking the medication,

- recent onset of substance abuse,
- ensuing mood disorder such as anxiety or depression.

20. Take care of yourself
- It is OK to get away.
- It is OK to get personal, marital, or family counseling.
- Do you or your spouse have undiagnosed or untreated ADHD or other mental health issues such as depression?

Homework Tips for Parents

A. Environment
1. Quiet, nondistracting. No TV. Soft music permissible. No cell phone or electronics.
2. All necessary tools available.

B. Timing
1. Best time after school, before dinner, e.g., come home → snack → unwind (play briefly) → homework.
2. If it is evening, finish 30 min before bedtime to "unwind."
3. Limit the total time to 2 h (if it takes longer, then negotiate with school to limit assignments).
4. Give a short break (3–5 min) every half hour (use a timer).

C. Being prepared
1. Get weekly homework assignment sheets in advance.
2. Use calendar to know when larger projects are due.
3. Use Homework Hotline (if available) to confirm assignments.
4. Consider using a cell phone to photograph assignments written on class blackboard.
5. School (or parent) to provide extra set of books at home (in case student "forgets" to bring home necessary books).
6. Have phone number of a peer available if needed to clarify an assignment.
7. PEARL: If child has ADHD, it is best to have medication onboard for homework time (it is difficult to do if student engages in sports after school, or procrastinates until late evening to start, because medication might cause insomnia).

D. Getting it done
1. Reward, e.g., finish homework → TV time.
2. Lots of praise for work completed.
3. Use incentives rather than nagging.
4. Do not feel the need as a parent to correct all errors (let the teacher do that).

5. If child has significant problems understanding how/what to do discuss with the teacher.
6. If necessary read or review instructions with child before he/she starts.
7. Divide homework into smaller segments with "mini goals."

E. Other helpful aides
1. Have a "homework buddy" (peer), preferably one who does not have ADHD.
2. Hire a "homework tutor" to come to the home, or the child can to go to an educational agency (private) for homework tutoring.
3. May even hire an upperclassman to be a homework tutor.

F. Utilize school services
1. Go to homework club after school (if available).
2. Attend a study skills class, e.g., at school, or through an outside agency such as Learning Disabilities Association, Sylvan.

G. PEARL: Arrange a 504 plan to provide, for example,
1. shortened assignments;
2. "grace period," e.g.,
    24 h for homework, in case it was done but "forgot to turn it in,"
    3- to 5-day "grace" for longer assignments and projects;
3. permission to dictate (vs. writing) or give an oral report privately to teacher for some assignments to decrease stress and time spent;
4. school to communicate (via phone, email, etc.) what homework is missing on Friday (or by Homework Hotline).

H. Ensuring completion and turning it in
1. Use "tough love" approach.
2. Withhold privileges/activities for the weekend until any and all assignments reported missing by the school on Friday are completed and signed off by a parent.
3. Place all completed work in the backpack the night before to ensure it is not left behind the next day.
4. Have a "fail-safe" system to ensure that the student actually takes it out of the backpack and turns it in, e.g., wrist watch alarm or cell phone notice.
5. Keep a running checklist of all the assignments
- when completed
- when turned in, etc.

These recommendations are summarized from Teenagers with ADD/ADHD (Chris Dendy) and The ADHD Book of Lists (Sandra Rief).

Index

Note: Page numbers followed by "f" indicate figures, "t" indicate tables.

Printed in the United States
By Bookmasters